T5-CVS-863

MEDICINE AND ANTHROPOLOGY

NUMBER XXI OF
THE NEW YORK ACADEMY OF MEDICINE
LECTURES TO THE LAITY

MEDICINE AND ANTHROPOLOGY

LECTURES TO THE LAITY, NO. XXI

THE NEW YORK ACADEMY OF MEDICINE

Iago Galdston, M.D., Editor

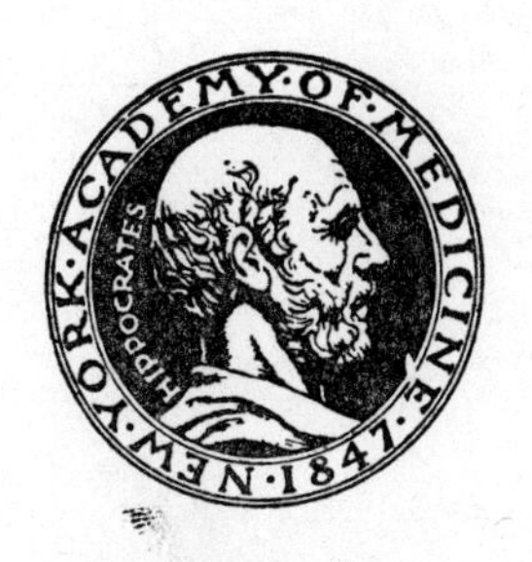

INTERNATIONAL UNIVERSITIES PRESS, INC.

NEW YORK 1959

The Committee on Laity Lectures in 1955-1956 was composed of Harold B. Keyes, M.D., *Chairman,* William H. Cassebaum, M.D., Waldo B. Farnum, M.D., Arthur M. Fishberg, M.D., I. H. Goldberger, M.D., Robert W. Laidlaw, M.D., Gervais W. McAuliffe, M.D., Harry Most, M.D., Thomas C. Peightal, M.D., Nelson B. Sackett, M.D., and Iago Galdston, M.D., *Secretary*

Library of Congress Catalog Card Number: 59-10378

Printed in the United States of America
By Hallmark Press, Inc., New York

CONTENTS

INTRODUCTION

By Iago Galdston, M.D.

ANTHROPOLOGY, understood in its literal sense, is the science of man. In that sense medicine must in effect prove an important component of anthropology. And so it is. But the converse is also true, and anthropology is, or should be, a significant component of medicine. Currently, however, it is not. Or rather, it is not commonly nor widely recognized as such. Some few among the medical specialists—psychiatrists, anatomists, haematologists, and immunologists—do find certain anthropological data pertinent to their special interests. But, in the main, anthropology is a *terra incognita* to most medical men and is not included in the premedical or medical curriculum.

In part, this is so because anthropology is comparatively young as a formal discipline—little more than a hundred years old. But this is not the whole reason. There are other disciplines just as young, or younger, which have been absorbed into medicine—biometrics, for example. The neglect of anthropology is more likely due to the fact that it is commonly taken to be the science of *ancient* man. Anthropology is equated to archaeology, the study of antiquities, and it is the vaunted conceit of modern science, medicine included, that it can learn but little from the ancients. This conceit is, of course, not entirely unwarranted. Modern science can learn but little that is *new* by studying that which is old. The texts of Democritus throw little light on the unsolved riddles of the atom. But there is much that is old which remains highly relevant to the new. This is less true perhaps for the physical sciences—physics or chemistry—but it is entirely true for the social and biological sciences, and in particular for medicine. Besides, while archaeology is a subspecialty of anthropology, it is not the equivalent of anthropology. In this relation the functional rather than the semantic definition of anthropology is to be preferred. In this version anthropology has the meaning of "the science of man and his works." This spells out the quality of a continuum. It relates the past to the present, or, more precisely, the present to the past, for no matter how new this brave world may be it is bound to and is buttressed by all that came before. Nowhere is this more patent than in medicine; in hygiene, in nutrition, in the rituals of doctor-patient relations—patent if one but looks to see.

This, I take it, is the burden of the first essay in this series, contributed by Dr. Paul Fejos, who is both physician and anthropologist.

It is of interest to observe that in times past it was not uncommon to find many physicians vitally interested in anthropological pursuits, not entirely as a hobby, but rather because such pursuits were pertinent to their medical concerns and interests. The name that comes to mind first is that of Virchow, the founder of cellular pathology, but there were many other physicians who were also anthropologists of stature. Among the better-known we may list Huxley, Haeckel, John Beddoe, Sir William Gull, C. E. Brown-Séquard, Pierre Paul Broca, L. A. Bertillon, Cesare Lombroso. It is interesting, and significant, that all these belong to the 19th century; not that there are not some medically trained anthropologists at work today. But, with few exceptions, these are primarily anthropologists, and not, as their precursors were, physician-anthropologists. The point I want to make is that toward the end of the last century medicine, largely under the impact of bacteriology, suffered a constriction in its interest and concern. It became much less of a humanistic pursuit and more of a scientific-technologic discipline. It learned a great deal more about a great deal less; it became less concerned with man and his works and more preoccupied with man and his diseases. That in narrowing its encompassments and in focussing its efforts on resolving the mysteries of disease causation, medicine did in effect achieve phenomenal results cannot be doubted or denied. And all that was for the good of man, and new. But, with the passing of time and the accumulation of collateral experience, it became evident, at least to some of the more perceptive, that medicine's preoccupation with disease causation, prevention and treatment, did not fulfill the larger expectations implicit in a true science of man and his works. It became apparent to those who looked beyond the immediacies of diagnostic, therapeutic and preventive measures, that man's well-being, his diseases, and his recoveries involved and depended upon other factors besides those embraced in the *science* of medicine.

In the early decades of this century men of earnest and penetrating thought began to advance new concepts, summated in such novel terms as homeostasis, medical ecology, holism, and psychosomatic medicine. These were essentially anthropological concepts, even though their labels were newly-coined terms—neologisms. Two disciplines served to marshal these *tentatives* into some order of structured meaningfulness. They were dynamic psychiatry and sociology. Psychiatry so to say rediscovered archaic man—finding him to be very much indwelling in the contemporary person. Sociology, taking its start at the communal perimeter, found much profit and instruction in the study of "the works of man." Their separate efforts have had the joint effect of revivifying the awareness that neither contemporary man, nor contemporary society, can be understood or effectively served save as they are studied in the perspectives of their long history. Such study *is* anthropology.

It is in this awareness and persuasion that The New York Academy of Medicine, with the generous support of the Wenner-Gren Foundation for Anthropological Research, organized the series of Laity Lectures here published under the title of *Medicine and Anthropology*. The nature and quality of this series of coordinate presentations is mirrored in the pre-eminence of the contributors. To Dr. Paul Fejos of the Wenner-Gren Foundation, Professor Marston Bates of the University of Michigan, Professor F. S. C. Northrop of Yale, Professor Alexander N. Leighton of Cornell, Professor Raymond W. Firth of the University of London, England, and Professor John W. Dodds of Stanford University, the Academy is deeply beholden. To Dr. Paul Fejos we owe a special debt of gratitude: Without his enthusiastic support, his guidance, and his multiform help this book "would not have been."

MAN, MAGIC AND MEDICINE

By Paul Fejos, M.D.

I HOPE you will allow me to try to define to some extent the word anthropology. It may seem superfluous; however, as a physician who has turned anthropologist, I have met some erroneous beliefs which I would like to put right.

In the less informed lay circles, we anthropologists are known as a queer group of individuals who for some esoteric reason love to handle smelly old skulls and greatly enjoy the company of murderous cannibals. There is also a somewhat more reasonable section within this group, the archaeologists, who are busy with a more profitable occupation, the search of the "lost" treasure of Incas or Mayas reputedly worth a king's ransom.

In truth we do little of this. Let me assure you that no archaeologist is happy when his misfortune brings him into contact with buried gold or jewelry. He, strangely enough, is much more enthusiastic upon encountering potsherds or a shell heap. Similarly the ethnologist is little interested in romantic derringdo or in cannibal raids, but finds great joy in recording the form of children's cradles or laboriously reconstructing the family tree of a primitive clan. In short, we believe that romantic adventures on a field trip are to be avoided. They are the result of bad planning of an expedition rather than personal courage and excellence.

What we do or attempt to do is signified by the name of our discipline. Anthropology, literally translated from the Greek, is the science of man. In all English-speaking countries the term is taken to mean "the science of man and his works." In Europe the term has been given a somewhat different meaning, being limited to the study of man's physical characteristics. As Linton said: "Anthropology differs from sciences like zoology, botany, physiology or genetics in one important respect. These sciences concentrate upon phenomena of certain limited sorts wherever they occur in nature. Anthropology has concentrated its interest upon a single organism: Man, and tried to understand all sorts of phenomena as they affect him. It has attempted to find out all that is to be known about this curious biped and his still more curious behavior" (1).

At present the main divisions of anthropology could be classified, somewhat arbitrarily, into: physical anthropology, the study of man's physical characteristics; and cultural anthropology, composed of linguistics, archaeology and ethnology. Archaeology deals with the beginnings of culture and with those cultures or phases of culture which are now extinct. Ethnology deals with the ways of life of societies which are still living or so recently extinct that fairly complete records are available.

I have used the word "culture" before. Let me define now what I mean by it. I use "culture" in its anthropological meaning. For anthropologists, "culture" is an important word. It does *not* mean what the German *"Kultur"* means: a learnedness, a sophistication, that is to say that a person can play the piano, and read the poems of Browning, and profess to like the paintings of Picasso. Culture for the anthropologist denotes the sum total of *socially* inherited characteristics of a human group. Thus culture comprises everything which one generation can tell, convey, or hand down to the next, in other words, the *non*-physically inherited traits we possess. We believe that man is distinguished from all other animals by the possession of culture. It is because he can speak, thereby frame ideas for himself and others of his kind, and because he can invent symbols, that he has culture, that he is human.

Today, our culture in Western society is incredibly complex. Compared to non-literate, primitive cultures, our socially transmissible body of knowledge, particularly in the field of natural science, is staggering to any imagination. It also shows, by contrast, the kind of culture man has had for maybe a million years. Some people call that period man's "animal-like" existence. I believe this to be a misnomer, because our ancestors, let's say in Europe's paleontological period, had brains as good as our own, but differed very much from animals by their possession of *culture*. Thereby they have known and were conscious of the precariousness of life and the inescapable fact of death. Thus they knew the worst of all constants, that all living organisms are sentenced to death when they are born. This must have made man's life bitterly harsh—a life constantly charged with the fear of disease and death.

Thus primitive man, ever since the earliest period of history, when face to face with bodily pain or mental anguish, or in danger of losing his life, must have sought salvation from some power *outside* of himself.

This brings us to another word I propose to define in its anthropological sense: magic. Contrary to its general use, the word "magic" does not denote trickery, prestidigitation or pulling out a white rabbit from a hat. Webster's dictionary defines magic as: "The art, or body of arts, which claims or is believed to be able to compel a deity or supernatural power to do or refrain from doing some act or to change temporarily the order of natural events, or which claims or is believed to produce effects by the assistance of supernatural beings, as angels, demons, or departed spirits, or by a mastery of secret forces in nature. Magic is not clearly differentiated from science by primitive peoples. It is a part of most primitive religions. With the rise of Christianity to power many magical practices were banned; the Church condemned resort to spirits and demons for knowledge or assistance (as in witchcraft, sorcery, diabolism) not as false, but as evil or *black magic.* Magic which aims to produce death or injury is also called *black magic.* On *white or natural magic* no ban was placed, and largely from this, which also survives in legerdemain, was developed modern natural science."

Magic means all the formulas for doing things which are beyond one's personal powers. It is not, however, a complicated proposition such as nuclear chemistry. It makes use of fairly simple things: *medicines,* which are the proper things to use, and *spells,* which are the proper things to say. Magic is world-wide. It is the property of *all* the *genus homo.* It is a fallacy to believe that magic exists only for the primitive. It exists for us as it existed for our ancestors. I hope to illustrate and prove this contention a bit later.

In Western society, magic is quite disreputable, but it has no bad reputation among primitive peoples. It is not a superstition or stupid belief for them, but is considered simply the right way of doing something. It is hardly possible for a primitive to define magic at all, or to see it as something by itself. For us Westerners, it is possible because we have developed the concept of science.

Curiously enough, there is a similarity between magic and science, in that people use science and magic to reach the same goals; but the basic philosophical assumptions of magic are different. Science accepts no compromises, nor contradictions, nor beliefs. Science wants to know if a thing or method will work, and why. Magic also wants to know whether a thing or method will work and is also much interested in the "why"; but it is willing to *believe* why, and does not look for physical reasons or causes. The causes, therefore, remain based upon faith and the supernatural.

Black magic is the most well-known. Over-all fear of black magic may be responsible for this. Black magic is the evil magic, the one used to kill, maim, render people impotent or sterile. White magic, on the other hand, always combats black magic, counteracts it, defends against it, neutralizes it. Amongst primitive people much more white magic is performed than black.

Magical practices are of four types: (1) *Sympathetic magic,* based upon the principle that like effects produce like results, or that a desired result may be brought to pass by mimicking it, naming it in spells, etc., and on the belief that things once in contact continue to act upon each other after being separated; (2) *Divination,* the various means of gaining hidden knowledge, as augury, clairvoyance, necromancy, astrology, etc.; (3) *Thaumaturgy,* or wonderworking, including alchemy and trickery ascribed to demons, etc.; (4) *Incantation,* the recital of magical formulas or pronouncement of a word or words of magical power or the performance of a magical ritual procedure.

Black magic is universally feared, not only in primitive societies but equally well in our own Western societies. Knocking on wood, not walking under a ladder, not seat-ing 13 at a dinner table—all such practices, that we call superstitions, are magic.

Magic is *honest*; that is to say, those who practice it believe in it. It is fully and unquestionably *valid* for them. Here lies, I believe, the basic obstacle to the average Westerner in viewing magic in its proper sense. For a Westerner, to knock on wood is a superstition; but to see a vaudeville act of sawing a woman in two is magic! The opposite is the truth! For in sawing a woman in two, the magician knowingly and with intent practices deception; he "tricks" his audience. The intentions of primitive magic, on the other hand, are never deception or trickery, but are rather based upon fully honest, dogmatic belief and faith.

Protective, white magic is used to insure us against black magic. The origins of many of these practices go back into the early history of man, but not all of them. White magic, particularly, is frequently born in modern societies, for instance, the belief that it is bad luck for three men to light their cigarettes from the same match. This arose in the First World War from magically logical reasons.

Possibly the ingroup-outgroup behavior pattern has its origin in the fear of black magic. Black magic as a rule can be practiced only extra-clanwise, the shaman of a clan being able to provide only white—protective—magic within his own group. His ability to do bad, black magic, is potential only toward the outgroup. Much of this belief still exists in our present-day society.

How is black magic practiced? The methods are astronomical in number. Libraries have been written about this, even in Western societies. Basically, the method seems to be to do things the "wrong" way, that is to say, backward, in the wrong order, the "bad" way, at the wrong time, with bad, malicious intent, for evil purpose. For example, in medieval times, the ill-famed "Black" Mass was a mass said backwards. It was said at night, and the consecrated host was black, not white. It was not round but angular, with three or seven points. It was not wine but water which the priest used for transubstantiation, and the water had to have had a bad history, such as water taken from a polluted well into which a newborn, but unbaptized, infant was thrown to drown.

In most primitive societies anything connected with the person against whom black magic is to be practiced can be used to make an effigy. This is the so-called "image" magic. Nail cuttings, hair, spittle, menstrual blood of a person are the best materials, but even belongings, such as wearing apparel, bedding, tools, weapons can be used. One method of using them would be for the sorcerer to fashion a figure representing the victim, using his saliva mixed with clay. If a lock of the victim's hair is available it is attached to the figurine's head, nail parings to its hand, and so on. Once the figure is finished, pins or thorns are stuck into it periodically. This process is accompanied by incantations of a definite traditional form. The incantations may be partly mumbo-jumbo, but they will usually contain words denoting the intent of the sorcerer. As the pins or thorns are stuck into the body of the figurine, the victim sickens. Sometimes, when the victim is aware that sorcery is being practiced against him, the corresponding parts of the body sicken or become paralyzed. Then the victim becomes ever more sick, and when, after several days or weeks, the sorcerer pierces the figurine's heart, the victim dies.

You will notice I said, "when the victim *is aware* that black magic is practiced against him." It is rarely the case that the victim does not know of the process. People love to talk and gossip in primitive societies just as much as in ours. The sorcerer will very likely visit the victim, or at least visit his dwelling, and may loiter about in the vicinity. In most instances the sorcerer himself announces that he is doing the evil magic as a "public relations" gesture to increase his social status in the community. There are records in Papua of a number of instances when a sorcerer, though actually innocent, confessed to the killing of victims to gain reputation. The sorcerer in most cases risks little in his own society, as to kill the sorcerer would be to no avail. One cannot *kill* magic. The fluid magic, the *mana,* will proceed swiftly from the dead body into another chosen one, and the danger of evil magic will still be over the head of the victim. One can combat, counteract, or neutralize magic; one cannot *kill* it.

Now let's take this new word I have mentioned, *mana.* It is a Polynesian word denoting "fluid, transmissible magic." It means a kind of force or power which can be present in anything or anybody and by its very presence can endow that person or thing with supernatural qualities. Mana is not, however, a spirit. It has no will or purpose of its own. Mana can be supplied by various sources. It may come from gods or spirits, it may exist naturally, or it may be instilled by a correct ritual. It may be transmitted by laying a hand of a person possessing it onto the body of a novice, or it can be simply "willed" into another body.

A native on the Papuan coast may find a stone or a shell which is peculiarly shaped, or has an unusual color, or it may come his way in circumstances he deems peculiar, magical or supernatural. He will take his find home and possibly bury it in his garden, because he will believe it has mana. If he now gets an unusually good harvest, he will know he was right. The stone had mana. Or he may bring it into contact with his spear, and if the spear proves afterward to be extraordinarily speedy and exact in finding the target, he will decide *it* has mana. It is not the workmanship, niceness of balance or straightness of the spear that counts in this instance. If now a spearmaker turns out consistently superior spears, which seem to find their way to the target with unfailing accuracy, then it is the *maker* of the tool that has the mana. There is no difference in the mana which is in the spear, the maker of it or in its owner. Mana will simply endow each of them with magical excellence.

Though the real home of the mana is the Pacific Ocean, it is found widespread all over the globe. We in Western society have a good share of it, though, as with magic, we hate to acknowledge it by its name. Instead we might call it a keepsake, memento, or simply our pet gun or tennis racquet.

During my travels in the United States I have encountered, in numerous houses, shiny silver dimes in elaborate frames. They are always hanging in a conspicuous place on the parlor wall. They were dimes received from John D. Rockefeller, Sr. by the father or the grandfather in the household. It seems Mr. Rockefeller frequently gave dimes to policemen, conductors or attendants. Curiously enough, none of these dimes were ever spent but were kept and highly treasured by the families of the recipients. They had the "Midas touch." Many of the owners told me that since the Rockefeller dime was in their possession, their families' material welfare miraculously improved. I must also mention that none of the owners of Rockefeller dimes whom I met seemed to be ashamed of harboring a "superstition," and most of them genuinely believed in the magical properties of the dime, as it had Mr. Rockefeller's magical touch.

The possession of mana, however, has its disadvantages. Chiefs, having close kinship with the gods, are usually endowed with much powerful mana. This can constitute an involuntary menace to others. Chiefs, kings and priests might have such powerful mana as to endow with fluid magic everything that comes into contact with their body. It is easy to see what can happen to a small kingdom—let's say an island in the Pacific—when a few generations of kings had walked on it. The land touched by the king's feet becomes dangerously potent with magic by that touch. In no time this can render an island sterile, because it becomes untouchable for an ordinary mortal. The carrying of kings and chiefs on ceremonial chairs and sedans may have its origin in this, as a protective measure. In primitive Polynesian philosophy mana must exist in a proper balance. Too much or too little is potent with disaster. Such upset in the equilibrium of mana is denoted by the Polynesian word *taboo.*

Taboo is something to be avoided because of an inescapable, unlimited danger for the transgressor. As with the word "culture," the anthropologist's meaning of taboo is different from its common usage. In common parlance it is taboo to eat baked beans with our fingers or to be guilty of any other breach of etiquette. I have even heard it said that it is taboo to park on the west side of Fifth Avenue. These are improper or unlawful, but not taboo. The supernatural is missing from them. One can park on the Avenue and get away with it, as the police may not come around. Breaking a taboo, however, will inevitably bring a horrible supernatural punishment upon the head of the transgressor and in some instances upon his family, clan and even upon his community. Such punishment is inescapable and inevitable. It may be impotence, sterility, failure of crop, disappearance of game, famine, or death. Transgression of taboo makes a person unclean, ritually bad, exposed to every kind of worldly or supernatural evil. Any and all transgressors of taboo are punished. One will bear the consequences if he breaks a taboo voluntarily or involuntarily. There is no recognition of mistake, accident, lack of malice. A transgressor is a terrible danger to his community. He is a supreme carrier of potential catastrophe—a veritable deadly Typhoid Mary.

All this should not, however, give you the idea that the natives live a dire existence, in eternal dread because of taboo. Rather, it should be viewed as an excellent system of signposts, showing the correct roads to take through all the phases of life from the cradle to the grave. The mere observance of a few limitations in diet, dress, work or behavior, ensures for the native the ability to look forward with confidence and tranquility to his future. It supplies a system of values to live by.

Now that the definitions of culture, magic, mana and taboo are out of the way, let us return to our subject: Man, Magic and Medicine. To man, be he Westerner or primitive, disease is a terrifying and abnormal state. It is potent with the ultimate of all disasters—death. To be able to return to a normal state we usually need help—help from someone who knows *what* our ailment is and *how* to combat it. That someone is the healer. In our Western society he is called the physician, the doctor, the M.D., or frequently that affectionate abbreviation, *Doc.*

In primitive societies also the healer has many names. We in Western culture call him witchdoctor, medicine man, sorcerer, magician, devil doctor. The anthropologist prefers the collective term: *shaman.* It is a Siberian word meaning one who is endowed with supernatural potentialities and abilities. Sometimes he is "possessed" by spirits. Both the physician and the shaman are learned men. Both of them are subjected to rigid discipline and a prodigious amount of education for many years. Both are under the rules of professional ethics. Both are usually respected members or leaders of their communities. In many primitive societies the shaman is also the priest. It is logical that he should be that, because of the primitive native concept of disease.

The rational, scientific concept of disease is a comparatively recent development in man's history. In immensely large areas of our world, even today, there is no such concept as "disease" in our sense of the word. Consequently there is no such thing as "natural," disease-caused death. For the primitive, "natural" death is the one caused by violence, accident, warfare, to be struck by lightning, to drown, to fall from a coconut tree. All other deaths are due to supernatural causes—magic. No matter how inconsequent, unreasonable or childish it may sound to you, it is for them, the primitives, the truth, the gospel, the dogma. It is not unreasonable to them, because their *reasoning* is different from ours.

There is no difference between the civilized, scientific physician and the shaman so far as their work or duties are concerned. They both will first endeavor to find the cause for the onset of the disease. They both take a history of the case (and let me tell those of you who ever complained that the doctor wasted your time with irrelevant questions as to which diseases you and your family had had, that a shaman taking a case history frequently spends hours and even days longer than his scientific colleague!) They both conduct and perform routine examinations of the patient's body. They both make a diagnosis and prescribe therapy. Frequently, too, they make a prognosis, an estimation of the future outcome of the ailment. Moreover, if the diagnosis is uncertain and "specialist" help is available, the shaman may call for consultation just as his colleague does in London, Paris or New York.

There is, however, a tremendous fundamental difference between the shaman and the physician in the concept of disease. As I told you, the native shaman is no trickster. He is just as honest and sure in his knowledge of the causes as his scientific colleague. But, whereas the province of the physician is anatomy, physiology and pathology—the natural sciences—the shaman's is magic, the supernatural. Hence it is easy to see that whereas the physician has his chemotherapy, his materia *medica,* his primitive confrère has his materia *magica.* The physician cures the patient through knowledge and understanding of the mechanism and functioning of the human body. The shaman works his therapy through the understanding of a supernatural world, very real and existing, but invisible and behind the real worldly scene.

The understanding of the supernatural world is the shaman's "scientific" knowledge. It was transmitted to him by his teachers much in the same way as our knowledge was instilled in us by our venerated professors in medical school. Furthermore, the truth of the supernatural was proved to him countless times during his apprentice years. He has seen for himself that the patients of his teachers were cured by them, made healthy again. He has had "experimental" proof that the theories taught to him are solid. The reasoning that the patients were cured is based on fact. No one will deny that. We westerners, however, object to the assertion that they were cured by the supernatural means used by the shaman.

How does the shaman cure an illness? The methods used all over the world would fill libraries and would be impossible to survey in the limited time I have. One could, however, somewhat arbitrarily, group the methods into three categories, according to the etiology of disease:

1. *Disease by intrusion of foreign objects.* Under this category fall all beliefs that a foreign object of evil power has entered the body of the patient, causing his illness. Such objects can be magical pebbles, small stones, thorns, arrows, miniature blowgun darts or even small living animals.

The therapy is obviously the removal of such object. This can be accomplished by the shaman's sucking the object out, squeezing it out with his fingers, forcing it out with tobacco smoke, with poultices or irritants, etc., or even enticing the object out by petting, stroking, tickling or fondling the diseased body.

2. *Intrusion by spirits or demons.* The patient's body has been entered into by an evil spirit or demon. These demons waste away the body of the patient because they eat up all the food he takes in. The spirit or demon, however, sometimes may not act as a true parasite and does not need any nourishment. In this case the ailment may be diagnosed—if the symptoms recur periodically—as the demon's "kicking up," making a row, in the patient's body. The treatment then will be the expulsion of the intruding spirit—exorcism. This can be accomplished mainly by ceremony, incantations, commands, or polite requests ad-

juring the spirit to depart, and not return. If the spirit does not respond, its temporary abode can be made unpleasant for it. This can be accomplished by making it "hot" for the spirit in a sweat bath, or freezing out the spirit by the application of cold. Some spirits will need to be starved out by a restricted diet or vigorous fasting. Demons sometimes depart if the diet is loathsome and disgusting. In such cases they can be expelled in a vomitus. A spirit can equally well be gotten rid of by cathartics. In some cultures, demons can be extracted by surgery, such as punctures or trepanations.

3. *Incidence of "soul capture" or "straying soul."* The patient's illness is caused by the absence of his soul. It is an AWOL proposition where the soul leaves the body without the owner's permission and enters into another sort of realm, or body, leaving the patient's body in distress, as the "chief" or "governor" of the body is absent.

The therapy here is to recapture the soul by ceremonial means and by making the patient's body attractive for it. The ceremonial means are usually incantations and the "locating of the soul." The latter is frequently a complex procedure of deductive reasoning, taking days or even weeks. The shaman, or his soul, becomes a sort of private eye for shadowing the straying soul. Dietary and hygienic measures are also ordered to make the body a desirable, comfortable home for the straying soul. If the patient's soul is captured with malicious intent by a sorcerer, then the power of that sorcerer needs to be fought, to give up the captive. This again is usually a long procedure, sometimes involving public duels between shaman and sorcerer.

The immediate causes for the onset of these "magical

ailments" can be: (1) *sorcery* or *black magic,* when a magic arrow is shot into the victim or a magic stone thrown into his body with malicious intent; image magic is practiced against him. (2) *sleep and dreams,* these are dangerous states. One is not in possession of all one's faculties. This is the most frequent onset for soul-straying. Particularly dangerous are dreams about illness or anything related to it. Most dangerous are dreams in which one violates a taboo. In such cases one may come under the next category, that of (3) a *ritually bad state or moral delinquency.* Here belong not only actual transgressions of taboos, but also careless execution of rituals or ceremonies. Diseases of such origin are always serious and the prognosis is at best uncertain. Patients afflicted with such ailments are usually on the shaman's critical list.

I have stated that primitive societies, where the disease concept is magical, have no materia medica, only materia magica. However, a number of important drugs and herbs, such as quinine, ephedrine and just now the Rauwolfia alkaloid, were taken over by western medicine from primitive societies. Thus my statement may seem paradoxical. An explanation may clear this up. If you visit a rubber plantation in Malaya, you find that the coolies of the plantation are paid a fee twice weekly to take the necessary prophylactic dose of anti-malarial medicine. It usually amazes the visiting Western tourist to find that the workers are paid for swallowing, for their own good, a medicament costing the plantation annually a large sum of money. But, from the coolies' viewpoint the atabrine or plasmochin is not a remedy. To them malaria is caused not by the presence of parasite plasmodium vivax in the blood, but by magical causes. Hence the white man makes the coolies swallow a bitter pill for no rational reason, but for his amusement or peculiar pleasure. It is right, proper and just therefore, that the coolies should receive payment for doing his bidding.

At the same time, if you would travel northward and visit a camp of the Bombay-Burma Teak Company in northern Siam, you will find native workers readily begging for anti-malarial medicines consisting of the same atabrine tablets, but given to them in conjunction with a complicated ceremony following a purification ritual and numerous dietary restrictions, certain clothing prohibitions and so on. Here the atabrine ceases to be a useless whim of the white man, but becomes a materia magica. It is therefore a logical therapeutic material to use.

In much the same manner most primitive medical practices contain—to borrow a sentence from television advertising—"medically proven active ingredients." In the Mentawei Islands, southwest of Sumatra, the standard therapy for diarrhea and dysentery is to send the patient at sundown to a certain point of the seashore, where he must lie down on the ledge of a white cliff and lie there flat and motionless for a definite period on his stomach and periodically lick the earth. The therapy is magical, but it has a scientific rationale nevertheless. The cliffs are a kaolin—a refined kind of clay—an absorbent which we frequently prescribe under the Latin name of *Bolus Alba.* It is a very effective medicine for diarrhea. The warm, sunbaked surface of the cliff acts as a hot water bottle or electric heating pad, and the psychosomatic effects of the shaman's mana frequently effect the cure.

Thus many of the facets of primitive medicine have a detectable scientific basis. Modern science, as a matter of fact, has some of its origins in it. The Indians of New England inserted a fish into each hill of corn they planted.

They taught this "magic" to the Pilgrim Fathers. They certainly could not have given any scientific explanation of enriching the soil with nitrogen. The Pilgrim Fathers, too, were ignorant of scientific theories of organic chemistry, but they followed the example of the Indians because they found it effective. Remember, magic is the formula of doing the right thing at the right time, using the proper thing and saying the proper words. Some of the "things" or some of the "words" become proper, in time, from experience with them. Thus many of the magical practices are based on empirical observations of natives. Once a thing consistently proves its superior excellence, it becomes endowed with mana.

On Soembawa Island, lives a shaman in the village of Do Dongo. Across his chest is tattooed a large circle with an ornamental capital letter B. He is my good friend and colleague, the shaman of the Dongo tribe. The story of his tattoo is a case in point. He was my principal informant in 1937 when I was doing field work on the ethnology of his tribe. We became fast friends through the several months of close association. He taught me native medicine and I occasionally helped out with his cases when he asked for my assistance or wanted me in consultation. All my drugs in the medicine chests originated from the German Bayer Company and on the packing cases was painted their trademark, an ornamented B in a circle. As I had taken all my "magical" supplies from such cases, my friend came to associate the power of my magic with the design of the trademark. After several months, he very formally asked my permission to use my magical symbol. As I have mentioned before, shamans are usually governed by very strict ethics. Less ethically, and without the permission of the Bayer Company, I released the copyright, and the letter B within the circle was emblazoned on my friend's chest. It gave him a tremendous additional amount of mana, and *de facto* increased his curative powers.

I am not being facetious about all this, and I ask you to realize that for the primitive concept of medicine these things are just as real and valid as our most cherished theories in serology or in the chemistry of the endocrine glands.

As a matter of fact, as mentioned at the beginning of this paper, magic is not the monopoly of the primitive people. We Westerners have our magical practices as well, though we label them as traditions or superstitions. When next you receive a prescription from your scientifically trained physician, remember that the RX on the top left corner is really an invocation to a deity for effective work of that prescription. I trust you will remember also that your physician's theories and knowledge are *not* based on magical theories, but on scientific facts. Nevertheless—though disappearing at a very rapid rate and with great acceleration—magic is still present in our time in our modern medicine. This is not "bad." It is an important adjunct and adjuvant to our chemotherapy, our surgery, our science, and above all to the art of medical practice. It is not trickery; it is not malicious intent to deceive.

Some time ago I attended a discussion in which physicians tried to determine what drug in the pharmacopeia is the most important and the most needed, the one without which medical practice would be unthinkable. My colleagues selected morphine and its derivatives as most important—the drug which enables the physician to allay pain speedily. I am tempted to offer the suggestion to add to it, magic. For without it, without the mana of the qualified physician, there would be no faith in the ability of the physician to heal—and only a physician could tell you how difficult, how almost impossible, it is to effect therapy in such a case.

This brings me to the last part of my lecture: the potential danger of not fully understanding the role of magic in medicine in general and particularly for the so-called primitive societies.

Our earth is shrinking in size with tremendous speed. Modern methods of transportation and communication are the reason. If the map of the world just before the travels of Columbus were represented as the size of a stage, that map has now shrunk to the size of a lectern. The steamship, the railway and now aerial transport by jet aircraft have made this so. The process we call civilization has made enormous, unbelievable inroads on primitive societies. Incredibly large segments of populations are subjected to civilizing processes by numerous methods of varying political and economic propaganda. Among these the public health reforms, based upon modern, scientific medicine loom large. It is of course well and proper that such reforms shall be effected, for it is an important organic part of programs of betterment for the backward areas.

The question uppermost in my mind is *how* far and by *what* means shall we effect the change? How much understanding and patience shall we need and exercise?

To illustrate my point: during World War II I lectured to officers and officer candidates of the Army and Navy who were being trained to act as liaison officers between the armed forces and primitive natives in the Pacific. The purpose was to prepare them for the possible eventuality of the misfortune that their arrival on a primitive island might coincide with the outbreak of a disease epidemic.

Such an occurrence is a great misfortune indeed, as the native population is likely to blame the newly arrived Western people for the outbreak of the disease, logically believing them to be evil magicians causing the disease. In my lecture I offered the suggestion to my students that if they should be confronted with such a situation, they should attempt to shift the blame away from themselves. As an expedient, I suggested that they put the blame on an animal, preferably a malformed one, or one of strange coloring, or to put it on a plant or a tree which had a strange appearance or location, and to devise a ceremony for removing that animal or object from the island and purifying the area where it was located. I gave prodigious numbers of suggestions as to how to make the ceremony properly complicated and impressive. At the end of the lecture, a young officer candidate, a Western-educated Korean, rose and in sharp words questioned the honesty of my suggestions. He pointed out that, instead of educating the natives, I was, with pernicious intent, fostering their stupid and barbarous beliefs, thereby leaving them in a dark state of ignorance instead of enlightening them. I asked this student what suggestion he would volunteer in such a case. Very matter-of-factly he told me that the natives should be told the truth, that the causative agent of cholera is the cholera vibrio Koch. I accepted his offer and asked him to use me as a native informant and give me the literal text he would deliver to a native. He launched into an explanation on the theory of micro-organisms, then abruptly stopped and said that he could not go any further without demonstrating the theory with a microscope. I then obtained a microscope from the biology department, together with a cholera slide which he put under the microscope and asked me to view the bacteria.

Acting out the native's role, I told him that I could see nothing, as of course no primitive native would be able to see through such a solid object as the ocular of a microscope, much less be able to recognize stained bacteria on a slide. About half an hour sufficed to convince my young Korean friend that it would indeed take months or possibly years to train a primitive native to use a complicated optical instrument, let alone to use it with understanding.

This may illustrate what difficulties a scientifically trained physician may encounter in a "magical" society. To inculcate concepts of bacteriology, pathology, physiology into the primitive mind will take time. Education is a very slow process even under ideal circumstances, and impatience and contempt for the natives' "stupidity" is not education—it is foolhardy folly which results in tragedy for educator and student alike. The process will need to be slow. It will need to be a slow transition rather than a fast change. We will need to adopt, temporarily, some of the native, primitive concepts in order to be able to educate.

How can such things be done? As in the case of the Bombay-Burma Company's anti-malarial campaign, magic will need to be part of the armament of modern medicine in such areas.

Some fifteen years ago I was doing ethnological field work among the Yagua, a little-known tribe located between the Amazon and the Putumayo Rivers in South America. My main informant was Unchi, the shaman, the most erudite and learned primitive physician I have encountered in some twenty years of field work around the world. We became very good friends during my stay with the Ant Clan, and I felt a deep sense of gratitude for the enormous amount of information he gave me, not only in the art of medicine among the Yagua but also on the customs and philosophy of his people. On some occasions he requested me to act as consultant on some of his cases. Mostly he wanted my aid whenever it was necessary to remove some of the teeth of his patients. Naturally I did the extractions under local anesthesia. For Unchi my ability to remove teeth painlessly was a highly impressive ceremony, and I believe he considered me and my instruments endowed with powerful mana. He also came to know that the magic of painlessness rested not in my forceps but in the dental syringe used for administering the anesthesia. It was logical for him to come to this conclusion, for the syringe received special ceremonial attention. It was taken apart, put into my portable sterilizer and vigorously boiled for a considerable time. Furthermore, my hands had been carefully washed and scrubbed before the components of the syringe were lifted from the boiling water. Unchi very quickly observed that once the syringe came out of the boiling water, it was handled with meticulous care. He came to know that once the instrument was sterile, it could not be touched and could not touch anything. The novocaine cartridges again were handled with a method which for him represented high magical ceremony, as they were carefully washed with alcohol and the solution gingerly extracted from them into the syringe. Unchi had witnessed these "ceremonies" possibly a dozen times. His eye never left my hands for even a fraction of a second, and he was in rapt attention throughout the process.

When the time came to leave the Yagua, I conducted the procedure, customary for ethnologists, of rewarding all my informants and distributing among the other members of the clan all such tools, wearing apparel and materials as we would leave behind. Partly in deference to Unchi's exalted position, and also out of gratitude and friendship, I asked Unchi before any one else to select whatever he would want from my belongings as a keepsake and reward for himself. I was almost sure that Unchi would want one of the *escopetas*. We had several of these muzzle-loading shotguns, which were very much admired and desired by the Yagua. Though they have splendid blowguns and curare-tipped darts, the range and effect of a shotgun meant much for Indians whose economy consists solely of hunting. Unchi, however, asked that I should part with my upper and lower root forceps, and my syringe. Without hesitation I handed over to him the two forceps, but—I am ashamed to say—I did not give him my syringe and store of novocaine. My refusal stemmed almost automatically from the belief that I could not put into the hands of an illiterate Indian an instrument for parenteral administration. I was afraid that possible lack of sterility, and ignorance in anatomical topography, might make the instrument in his hands a potential danger.

A few days after my departure on a wood-burning Amazon steamer, I had much idle time in which to reflect, and I wished that my decision in not giving Unchi the syringe had been better considered. I could have spent some time teaching Unchi how to sterilize the syringe, where to insert the needle and in what direction—all, of course, not on a scientific basis of germ theory and regional anatomy but simply as a highly potent magical procedure. Unchi would have learned fast and would have been more than qualified to execute the "ceremonies" with an unheard-of meticulousness and without error.

Any physician will bear me out that it is a difficult educational process to teach a student in a nursing school the importance of sterility in parenteral administration. Though the concept of micro-organisms is well inculcated in the student's mind, he or she is liable to slip, forget, when under pressure or tired. The sterility of a hypodermic needle thus may be questioned in the hand of a novice, though, fortunately, I believe rarely. It would never need to be questioned in the hands of my friend Unchi. His very life, his existence, his salvation, even his community's, would be at stake—not only his job or the welfare of a single patient.

Thus magic can be a potential ally of the scientific physician. Used with full understanding it can become one of his important tools, not only in education of primitives but also in the art of his practice, not as unethical trickery, not as malicious aid, but as a fully proper, rational, scientific adjunct for healing the sick.

REFERENCE

Linton, Ralph, ed.: *The Science of Man in the World Crisis.* New York: Columbia University Press, 1945, pp. 3-4.

THE HUMANIST LOOKS AT THE DOCTOR

By John W. Dodds, Ph.D., Litt.D.

IT MIGHT be well, right at the beginning, to establish my description of the humanities. It is a term that has been so variously interpreted, and has been attached to so many schools of thought, that one is sympathetic with the man in the street who identifies the humanities vaguely with humanitarianism in general, and equates the study of *Paradise Lost* with flood-relief. When we established a School of Humanities at Stanford University some years ago, one of the first letters we received was from the Society for the Prevention of Cruelty to Animals. Another came from a woman in San Francisco who said that she knew we would be sympathetically interested in her cause: she ran a lonely hearts bureau.

Although nothing human is really alien to the humanities, they do mean a little more than that. In university curricula, where labels tend to stick, they are usually identified with the creative or speculative side of man's activity —the literatures, arts, music, philosophy, drama, and the like. History plays a dual role; it partakes of the nature both of the social sciences and the humanities—although if what the dean of English historians, George Macaulay

Trevelyan, says, is true, that "history is an informed guess at the most likely generalization," then the scientific value of history becomes less evident.

In general, then, the humanities deal with the creative, imaginative side of man's nature as revealed in history, in great works of literature and art, and in the great philosophies. But as I understand the term they mean more than that, for they are, or should be, concerned with man's social as well as his spiritual environment. They differ from the sciences, and the social sciences as usually practiced, in their effort to find some kind of unity and significance in the phenomena of human life. They are concerned with everything that endows life with *meaning*. Therefore, they deal primarily with *values,* and their job is to interpret and evaluate the patterns of our existence, not so much in terms of conflicting ideologies or metaphysical systems—Aristotelian or Kantean or Lockean or Marxian —as in a much more personal and individual frame of reference. They are concerned with man—man living, breathing, acting, pounding out on the anvil of his little existence between two darknesses the ideals, the moral imperatives, the ecstasies and the disappointments, the victories and the defeats which torment and bless him.

To pin this down specifically, what does a major literary work, for example, really do for us? To begin with, it deals with universals, with human destiny—man's loves, hopes, and aspirations, as well as his doubts and despairs. Thus we learn about the common nature of men, and our sense of identification with others is heightened. A great book or play does this not in terms of abstractions, but by revealing character in action—not jealousy, but Othello; not irresolution, but Hamlet. Such is the nature of the artist's insight that we discover the Othello and the Hamlet in ourselves; we are led toward self-understanding. We learn that character counts. If an author creates a man or woman with a certain moral bent, then the actions in which that person engages will have certain inevitable consequences. There is a law of cause and effect in human nature as well as in external nature.

Moreover, a great book raises problems that reach beyond it. What is the relation between man's freedom and his responsibility? Our basic democratic assumption is that man, however much his career may seem to be determined by heredity or environment, *has* freedom of choice. It is that which gives him dignity and importance. Science may prove that man is relatively weak and insignificant, that what seems to him his freedom is so limited that even equality of opportunity becomes a sterile fiction. Great literature, on the other hand, demands the recognition of the worth of every human being, however much he may appear to be hemmed in by circumstance or the victim of his own genes. Thus literature supports by *insight* those axioms of our democracy which are, at bottom, also matters of insight—for the dignity of man is not susceptible to measurement.

A great work of art, then, teaches us that responsible choices are important, teaches us how to live, teaches us morality in Matthew Arnold's broad sense, "the application of ideas to life." It does not do this didactically; it operates by example rather than precept. Shakespeare does not say anywhere in *Macbeth,* as I remember it, that too much ambition leads to horrible results, or in *Lear* that hot-headed, foolish old men are likely to get into trouble. But the meaning is clear.

There is one thing more that a major work of literature can do for us: it can give us courage to face life as it is, not as we should wish it to be, and thus teach us to think more compassionately and more hopefully of our fellow men and more courageously of ourselves. It is not that a hero in a Shakespearean tragedy, for example, is "successful" in any ordinary sense of the word. Buffeted by fortune, confounded by the dark recesses of his own nature, sinking at last in the maelstrom horrors which overwhelm him, he goes down at last in seemingly catastrophic defeat. Yet it is not all defeat. In the midst of tragedy, the measure of man is not his final capitulation to the forces which annihilate him; it is the temper with which he meets those forces. And it is the glory of literature to affirm spiritual victory in the midst of physical defeat, and to enable us to sense, even as all seems lost, the triumphant invincibility of the human spirit which can rise above disaster. Thus we are made able to understand that men, in their potential, are

> One equal temper of heroic hearts,
> Made weak by time and fate, but strong in will
> To strive, to seek, to find, and not to yield (4).

If literature can do this for us, why should it be treated as a luxury, and science as the only necessity?

It is perhaps in their creative aspects that the humanities best express these tough and stubborn truths, but to limit the humanities thus severely is to distort them. Nothing is more artificial, for example, than the distinction between the humanities and the social sciences—except perhaps in the case of the newer mathematicians who are searching currently for formulae which will pin down in a series of *x*'s and *y*'s all social and artistic human achievement. (When this happens, we might as well let Univac take over.) But in general, the social sciences and the humanities should be in each other's laps. As soon as you begin to *interpret* as well as to collect statistical data, you are in the main stream of the humanities. There is a humanistic way of looking at science (just as there can be an unhumanistic way of teaching Shakespeare). In general, sympathy and understanding are the goals of the humanist—an understanding of the rich texture of man's personality and achievement, and a compassionate appreciation of the subtle but profound complexities of his lonesome career.

If I were to lead you in advance to my conclusion, therefore, it would be that every medical man should be—must be—a humanist. But how do we get to that point? It will take some doing.

The practice of medicine is still pretty much of a mystery to most people—although not so much, perhaps, as it was before the newspapers and magazines began telling us what we ought to ask the doctor to prescribe. But at the very least there is a morbid fascination about this subject. (Few novels written about medical subjects have failed.) The doctor is still something of a magician, a medicine man in the primitive sense. Witness how much credibility the mere donning of a white jacket gives to any television announcer whose duty it is to declare the biological merits of a new toothpaste!

Because of this mysterious lure—and because, too, of the responsible and influential place the physician holds in modern society—the status of the doctor today is higher than at any time in our history. Surveys show that if you ask parents what profession they would like their children to enter, the medical profession leads all the rest. As a friend of mine has pointed out to me, this was not always so. If you had asked a parent in the eighteenth century in this country what he would most like his boy to become, he might well have said: "a minister." There was no more socially desirable profession. Later on in the century, after the Revolution and the construction of the new United States, it would have been the law. In the nineteenth century, when the Industrial Revolution was really being felt—and the legal profession seemed to many people what it seemed to Thomas Carlyle: "a shapeless mass of absurdity and chicane"—the parent would have wished his child to be an entrepreneur in big business, a captain of industry. Later on the banker came into his own; he manipulated the fortunes which the businessman accumulated, and the ideal of every Alger hero was to become a banker. Well, we all know what happened to bankers in the 1930's. And today, the medical man sits on top of the heap. I draw no parallels from the earlier cyclic history of the professions except to point out that statuses *have* sometimes changed!

Along with the emerging prestige of the doctor has come the phenomenal advance of medical knowledge in our generation. Some time ago I was interested in exploring the decade of the 1840's, in England, and it was appalling to realize how primitive medical science was merely a hundred years ago. Ether anesthesia was first introduced in 1846. In 1849 a devastating scourge of asiatic cholera hit England, and the only remedies available to the medical profession ranged from the use of calomel and tartar emetic to packing the patient in a wet sheet and feeding him three small cups of olive oil. The best authorities favored the "zymotic" theory of the disease: that cholera arose from the swamps and was carried by atmosphere impregnated with "pestilential miasmata." It seemed to worry few people that all the London sewers—sixty of them—emptied into the Thames, whence six of the nine water companies drew their supplies of water for the metropolis. Two thirds of the companies had no system of filtration. This was the situation well into the reign of Queen Victoria. The wonder is, not that so many died, but that anyone lived! Medical histories point out that as a whole the treatment of disease in the early nineteenth century was hardly more advanced than in Hippocratic days.

Certainly the recent advance of medicine has been fantastically rapid, even though today all the skill of the profession could do nothing about a disease which attacked me the last time I visited New York City. Doctors could tell me that it was caused by one of the smaller viruses, about 60 millimicrons across, for which there was no treatment but aspirin and taking to one's bed. I refer, of course, to the common cold. We know so much, and we know so little!

Now what has been medicine's historic connection with the humanities? More in the past, I venture to say, than in the present. Hippocrates, who seems to have been a pretty hardheaded clinician, always speaks of the "art of medicine," and the Pythagoreans used music as well as medicine to cure the ill. "Art," to Hippocrates, may have included what we call "science," but today one speaks only of "medical science," and the change is both significant and symptomatic. In its early days, medicine was closely associated with what we know now as philosophy—the worse for ancient medicine, perhaps! The medical theory of the four humors, of the Hippocratic physicians and of Galen, the theory which dominated the Middle Ages, was a philosophical theory of disease: any imbalance in the humors generated disease. The great Renaissance physician, Paracelsus, demolished witheringly the theory of the humors and turned chemistry loose on the analysis of disease. But he himself was highly speculative and fed upon a kind of fantastical mysticism. Even after the time of Harvey, medical theorists tried to establish complete systems which were more metaphysical than scientific. And in our own generation, Freud's detailed and systematic observations became for him the basis of an elaborate set of speculative theories which not all his followers were able to tolerate.

Doctors no longer exorcise demons, but philosophy, or superstition (if it's philosophy you don't believe in) has always been the handmaid of medicine. When Apollonius was called to treat a woman in the throes of a difficult labor, difficult because of her narrow pelvis, he told the anxious husband to take a live rabbit and walk around the woman with it. "This single sample of his medical activity," writes one medical historian, "is sufficient to characterize Apollonius as a charlatan of the most contemptible class." I wonder. I don't know what Apollonius could have done about the narrow pelvis, and I suspect that the therapy did no harm. It might even have quieted the husband and thus have given some comfort to the wife!

Among primitive tribes, as Dr. Fejos told you in an earlier lecture, medicine is mixed up with sorcery and witchcraft, depending upon amulets, charms, taboos, and noxious potions—their particular appeasement of demonic forces. But sound therapy, evolved through who knows what ages of trial and error, sometimes went hand in hand with pure superstition. Modern medicine discovered important drugs in common use in primitive cultures, such as the cinchona of the Peruvian Indians, and the curare of the Amazon. Primitive peoples, from the Papuans to the Africans to the Indians of the United States, have always used steam and vapor baths for rheumatic pains. Massage was a standard therapy in Melanesia, intended to drive the malicious spirits from the body; but whatever the theory of disease might be, the results are the same as in modern physiotherapy!

Perhaps the best-known doctor-philosopher-humanist in the range of English letters is the incomparable Sir Thomas Browne, who quietly practiced his medicine during the lifetime of William Harvey, but is known today for his beautiful statement of his philosophical principles in *Religio Medici* (1643); for his curious study of "vulgar errors," *Pseudodoxia Epidemica* (1646), where he examines the natural history of unicorns and glow-worms; and for his *Hydriotaphia; Urn-Burial, or a Discourse of the Sepulchral Urns Lately Found in Norfolk* (1658). Sir Thomas's beautiful, majestic prose has made him one of the enduringly great English stylists.

Listen to him speaking in *Urn Burial* of the fickleness of self-perpetuation:

"What song the sirens sang, or what name Achilles assumed when he hid himself among women, though puzzling questions, are not beyond all conjecture. What time the persons of these ossuaries entered the famous nations of the dead, and slept with princes and counsellors, might admit a wide solution. But who were the proprietaries of these bones, or what bodies these ashes made up, were a question above antiquarianism; not to be resolved by man, nor easily perhaps by spirits, except we consult the provincial guardians, or tutelary observators. Had they made as good provision for their names as they have done for their relics, they had not so grossly erred in the art of perpetuation. But to subsist in bones, and be but pyramidally extant, is a fallacy in duration. Vain ashes which in the oblivion of names, persons, times, and sexes, have found unto themselves a fruitless continuation, and only arise unto late posterity, as emblems of mortal vanities, antidotes against pride, vainglory, and madding vices. . . .

"But the iniquity of oblivion blindly scattereth her poppy, and deals with the memory of men without distinction to merit of perpetuity. Who can but pity the founder of the pyramids? Herostratus lives that burnt the temple of Diana, he is almost lost that built it. Time hath spared the epitaph of Adrian's horse, confounded that of himself. In vain we compute our felicities by the advantage of our good names, since bad have equal durations, and Thersites is like to live as long as Agamemnon. Who knows whether the best of men be known, or whether there be not more remarkable persons forgot than any that stand remembered in the known account of time?"

Hear Sir Thomas declaring his physician's creed:

". . . Let me be sick myself, if sometimes the malady of my patient be not a disease unto me. I desire rather to cure his infirmities than my own necessities. Where I do him no good, methinks it is scarce honest gain; though I confess 'tis but the worthy salary of our well-intended endeavors. I am not only ashamed, but heartily sorry, that, besides death, there are diseases incurable: yet not for my own sake, or that they be beyond my art, but for the general cause and sake of humanity, whose common cause I apprehend as mine own. . . ."

Is the Hippocratic oath any better than that?

I reread the Hippocratic oath the other day, and was impressed again by the nobility of its ethical statements. But I was also impressed by how large, proportionately, was the space given to the responsibilities of the physician to his fellow-craftsmen in the guild of medicine. I notice, incidentally, that the sentence, "With purity and with holiness I will pass my life and practice my art" is omitted from the abridged form as given to modern graduates in medicine.

Medicine and Anthropology

I began this section by speaking of the transformation of medical art into medical science. I wonder, however, if medicine at its best, will not always be something of an art? Certainly a good diagnostician is an artist. What any artist does is to select, from the broad stream of human experience, what seems to him its significant aspects or moments, to recombine them and to fuse them, under the fire of his imagination, into a new synthesis which represents his vision of reality. What does the doctor do but this—analyzing symptoms, weighing appearances, combining them and fitting them into a pattern; and arriving, sometimes logically, sometimes with a burst of near-intuition, at an understanding of the typical or the atypical, and thus forming his diagnosis. Here is an act of the creative imagination of the highest order.

More and more, however, the "healing art" has become "medical science," until medicine is on the verge of becoming a technology. The multiple millions of dollars poured into medical research have resulted in profound benefits for suffering humanity. But the inevitable correlary to that is an emphasis upon the various specialties; the human frame and its illnesses have been charted and divided and subdivided; the increase in medical knowledge is such that no one man today can pretend to comprehend the whole. The result is the obsolescence (to speak in technological terms) of the general practitioner. What young medical student today wants to devote his life to the routine care of ordinary illnesses when all sorts of fascinating specializations, with correspondingly increased prestige and financial return, lie before him for the choosing? Here is a list of some of them: anesthesiology, dermatology, internal medicine, neurological surgery, obstetrics and gynecology, ophthalmology, orthopedic surgery, otolaryngology, pathology, pediatrics, plastic surgery, psychiatry and neurology, radiology, and urology. More and more today the patient tends to bypass the general practitioner and seek out the specialist who, according to the patient's self-diagnosis, is equipped to treat his illness. And such is the nature of the doctor, who is a human being, that, as the Final Report of the Commission on Medical Education of the Association of American Medical Colleges (1932) put it: "because his efforts are often confined to a single phase of medicine, the specialist looks too frequently upon the problem of the patient solely from the aspect of his specialty, rather than from the needs of the patient as a whole" (p. 24). The quandary is a real one, however, for medical knowledge is so gigantic that the doctor is forced to a division of labor.

We have paid a price for our knowledge. Impersonality does very well in electrical engineering; how about *human* engineering? Whatever pains I may have, I'm still a whole human being in terms of a total personality. Is it too much to ask the doctor to treat me as a human being, to find the person in the patient? I know that disease is a biological process, but to myself, at any rate, I seem like more than a bundle of biological responses. As such the prospect of push-button medicine frightens me. If a layman like myself wanted to construct a nightmare, it would be set in a long marble hall down which I passed, with my particular ache, on a moving belt. As I went by, machines would appear from nowhere to diagnose me. I would be palpated by an artificial hand; at various stations I would be x-rayed, ophthalmoscoped, stethoscoped, electrocardiographed and basally metabolized. Mechanically operated syringes would draw blood from me; a thermometer would be popped automatically in my mouth. And if I were to cry out with

Macbeth, "Canst thou not minister to a mind diseased, pluck from the memory a rooted sorrow, raze out the written troubles of the brain?"—I would be presented with a flash-card reading: "Pre-frontal lobotomy indicated." As I got off that moving platform I would wait until the electric calculating machine finished flashing and clicking, and at last I would pick out of a slot my prescription, accompanied by a blank check. This is a completely frivolous conception, of course. A proper nightmare would allow for the introduction of some sort of standardized "beside manner."

The problem of overmechanization, to be sure, is not peculiar to medicine; it is one of the saddle-sores of our age. Nothing is clearer than that our technology has outrun our sociology. Ever since steam was harnessed to machines, and the Industrial Revolution got under way, man's ability to control his physical environment has outstripped his ability to control himself. With the twentieth century the acceleration has become phenomenal, and the gap has gotten steadily wider. We ride the skies in supersonic splendor; we create marvels of technological ingenuity; we discover antibiotics so that we can make more people live longer, so that they can be run down by faster and faster automobiles; we extract the basic secrets of the atom so that we can explode ourselves into eternity by the millions rather than by the hundreds. We are the masters of the universe—and spiritually and ethically and sociologically we are still (comparatively speaking) crawling around in the primeval slime.

Now medicine shares in all this technological glory, and though its conception is still the physical salvation of mankind, it too has traps awaiting it. The Final Report of the Commission on Medical Education supports me here too: "[Efforts to standardize procedures] in medical services are based in many instances upon the fundamental fallacy that the human being, who is the unit of medical service, can be regarded as a uniform, standardized organism. Sound medical practice requires careful study of the health needs of each individual—physical, psychic, and social . . . Another tendency in medical practice is the emphasis placed upon mechanical devices . . . But the laboratory findings are valuable only in so far as they are correlated with the medical problem of a given patient" (3, p. 22). In other words, not merely what bacillus is invading me, but am I happy with my wife, is my job getting me down, am I worried about my debts, why do I accept invitations to give public lectures—things to which no laboratory can ever give an answer.

If the modern doctor is to fulfill his obligation to his patient, therefore, he will have to approach him with more than penicillin—with an understanding of the profound "importance and influences of social, economic, and psychological factors as they contribute to the causation, treatment, and prevention of disease in the individual" (3, pp. 64-65). The doctor must know more than medicine. He must be broadly cultured, able to understand life in all its phases. To the qualities of honesty and integrity he must add literacy, an awareness of the relation of men to their social and spiritual environment, a sensitiveness to man's imaginative accomplishments, and some knowledge of those accomplishments. He must be aware of the place of medicine in the total spectrum of man's knowledge. He must have the qualities of a good general practitioner; he must be a superb specialist; and in addition, he must be an educated man in the broad rather than the narrow sense. This is clearly a call for paragons, and paragons are hard to come by nowadays. It is only one's profound respect for the medical profession and awareness of the responsibilities of modern medicine, that gives one courage to insist upon such Renaissance men. At the very least, to treat the whole man, the doctor must be a whole man himself.

Now what should medical education do to produce such men? Certainly it should help the student to sense the social dimensions of the profession he is entering. If medicine is a form of public service he must be aware that the public will be interested in the kind of service it is getting—and that unless it gets adequate leadership from the profession it will itself try to move in and call the turns. More and more it is becoming evident to most people that civilized countries cannot afford to neglect the health and well-being of large portions of their entire populations, that effective medical services must reach everybody. The question is, how is this to be done? At this point I fear that the medical profession has spent much of its organized time throwing road-blocks in the path of progress. I am not referring now to that nasty idea "socialized medicine," (which I hope Americans will never have to endure) but rather to the program of organized medicine to brand as "socialized" the efforts, public and private, to create types of voluntary methods to distribute the spread of medical services and costs. A good friend of mine who is a doctor declares that if true state medicine were ever to come to America through the demands of a public frustrated in its groping for adequate medical care, the medical profession itself should be held mainly responsible.

A few years ago Dr. Raymond B. Allen wrote for this very Academy which I am now addressing a book called *Medical Education and the Changing Order*. Let me quote him on this point. "Physicians of the future," he writes, "must be capable . . . of viewing the problem of medical service dispassionately. Unless they recognize the right of every person to adequate medical service, the medical profession will degenerate to the level of a trade. . . . Has the medical profession up to this time shown the necessary social vision to cooperate with the community at large under both volunteer and public auspices in conceiving and carrying out programs for the improved distribution of medical services? In the sphere of the economics and sociology of medical care, looking toward a wider distribution of high-quality service, the profession as it expresses itself through its regular organizations has failed to meet some of its responsibilities to society. Medical education shares in the responsibility for the failure of the medical program to exhibit social insight and aggressive leadership in the problem of adequate medical care for all the people" (1, pp. 29, 30, 32). Allen goes on to point out that the organized profession opposed establishing satisfactory workmen's compensation laws; it opposed pre-payment insurance plans for hospital care; it opposed pre-payment insurance plans for professional services. "It did not show vigorous, imaginative leadership or social insight in its approaches to these problems. Rather, it tended to hold back until public pressure was such that it had to go along" (1, p. 30). Dr. Allen was writing in 1946.

I wonder what progress has been made in the last ten years on this front of educating the doctor? Knowing academic institutions and professional societies, and their resistance to change, I wonder what kind of education the medical student is getting today in these areas of public, as well as professional, concern. Are they merely being given more sand to stick their heads into?

There is another kind of *social* (not socialized) medicine which the medical student should be instructed in. If it is true that the study of medicine involves life in all its aspects, psychological and social as well as physical, then the emotional and mental life of the patient, together with his environmental life, becomes a matter for medical concern. Not to understand these stresses is to misunderstand the patient and to offer him partial and incomplete therapy. It involves preventive medicine in its most important frame of reference, not immunology, for to keep the patient well the doctor needs more knowledge than how to use the x-rays or toxoids of preventive medicine. It involves a knowledge of the patient in relation to his total environment. As Dr. Galdston so well points out in his book *The Meaning of Social Medicine,* it is not just immunology or public health or geriatrics; it is the consideration of total man in his total milieu, and should interpenetrate *all* branches of medicine—not merely in terms of health and disease, but in terms of life; "to sustain and improve well-being" (3, p. 82). Dr. Galdston calls it "eubiotic" medicine, "that is, medicine dedicated to help the individual to achieve the best that he is capable of in his experience in living" (3, p. 92). Here lies a great challenge for medical education, which at present I suspect, it but dimly perceives.

To be educated for this kind of service the student needs more than the conventional anatomies, histologies, physiologies, bacteriologies, diagnostics, therapies, etc., which have been his traditional curriculum. He needs these too, but he needs more. I am never surprised at the courses which medical schools prescribe for their students, but I am surprised at what they *fail* to prescribe, either as part of the medical or premedical curriculum. Psychiatry has at last crept in as an essential. But how about such a subject as cultural anthropology? This synthesizing science, dealing with the cultures of mankind and with many varieties of phenomena as they concern man, would seem very important for the medical student. Psychology, particularly social psychology, and sociology—these furnish an invaluable basis for the understanding of modern man. To the extent that medicine is a social science the premedical student must be brought in contact with these important disciplines. Present premedical curricula largely ignore them, or at least do not stipulate them.

In general, there is an imperative need for the liberalization of the premedical and medical curriculum. I have heard medical educators agree in conference and in conversation that the broadly cultured person makes the best medical student, but when it comes time to set up the requirements for entrance to schools of medicine all this seems to be forgotten. One medical school with which I am familiar lists 53 units of requirements in chemistry, physics and biology for its minimum admission requirement (it specifies no other courses except a year of freshman English composition). The announcement points out that such premedical requirements leave plenty of time for liberal electives. In the fine print, however, it "recommends" that students applying for admission should complete 21 additional units in biology and chemistry. In the competition for entrance to medical schools the student reads the fine print. Which would he choose, do you suppose, courses in anthropology and philosophy or more work in chemistry?

And if fledgling doctors need some sophistication in the social sciences, what about studies in the traditional humanities? Don't doctors need history, to enable them to see the present in the perspective of the past? Don't they need some minimum of philosophy and logic, to know how man conceives of himself and the universe? And don't they need to be brought face to face with the riches of literature and art, so that they can enter deeply into the imaginative experiences of others, and thus extend the scope of their own sympathetic understanding? It is here that they learn to value their own humanity and that of their fellow human beings. Here it is that they get the wisdom which the best minds have spoken through all the ages. Tennyson wrote: "Knowledge comes, but wisdom lingers," and if we ever needed wise people, we need them as doctors. The humanities deal with life and hope and fulfillment—life made rich and worthwhile. It is life which it is the doctor's task to conserve; not only the biological process, but the fullness of *living*.

I was pleased recently to come across the presidential address of Dr. Daniel C. Elkins (2) to the American Surgical Association. It was called "A Case for the Study of the Humanities in the Making of a Doctor." He quoted Alan Gregg, who said that the fruit of man's preoccupation with nature must "give way to Humanism, the flower of man's experience with man."

"If we concentrate our energies, our thinking, and our values only on atoms and hormones," Dr. Elkin went on, "then we have indeed left ourselves vulnerable to destruction by the very thing we seem to worship and seek to conquer." He urges the elimination of the word "premedical" from the curriculum. "If 'premedical' meant a sound and inspiring education in scientific and humanitarian thinking and an acquaintance with cultural achievements, so combined and so offered that the student is inspired to recognition of his own potentiality, then there would be no lost time and crossed purpose for the students who *do not* get into medical school; and those who *do* would have acquired a proper background of education. But I have just described what does not exist" (2).

The impractical professional humanist, living (supposedly) with his head in the clouds, sentimentally aware of the beauty in life but innocent of any sense of its demanding practicalities, is grateful for statements like these from quarters beyond suspicion.

I end, then, with the conclusion which I stated long ago in advance: every doctor should be—must be—a humanist. If I wish so much for the medical profession, concerning which I may have seemed sometimes to be severe, it is because I admire it so greatly, and share with most people today a keen sense of its dignity and importance, and wish for it nothing but the best in the new society which is always in the making.

REFERENCES

1. Allen, Raymond B.: Medical Education and the Changing Order. Cambridge: Harvard University Press, 1946.
2. Elkin, Daniel C.: A Case for the Study of the Humanities in the Making of a Doctor. *Ann. Surg., 136*:338, 342, 1952.
3. Galdston, Iago: *The Meaning of Social Medicine*. Cambridge: Harvard University Press, 1954.
4. Tennyson, Alfred Lord: *Ulysses*.

THE ECOLOGY OF HEALTH

By Marston Bates, Ph.D.

THE "ecology of health"—it sounds very elegant, but what does it mean? It's easy to check with the dictionary. Ecology: "biology dealing with the mutual relation between organisms and their environment." Health: "state of being hale or sound in body, mind, or soul." Putting these together, I take it that my topic for tonight is concerned with the environmental conditions favorable to a state of well-being—in body, mind and soul.

When I went through the dictionary operation, I was appalled at what I had undertaken. Separately, the two words seem harmless enough. "Ecology" in recent years has become one of the most frequently used words in my vocabulary. I like to think of myself as a naturalist rather than an ecologist, but I have gradually become reconciled to the learned sound of the Greek-root word, and I use it easily and frequently without flinching. As for health—I worked for seventeen years for the International Health Division of the Rockefeller Foundation, which gave me considerable opportunity to talk about health. I never quite understood what the word meant, but lack of understanding, of course, rarely prevents people from talking. If it did, I suppose we would all become Trappists.

Ecology and health, then, seem easy and familiar enough.

The trouble comes when we put them together. I shall feel safer if I deal with them separately for a while.

Ecology is a biological science. It is concerned with individuals, populations and communities and with the interactions of these with each other and with the environment. I like to think of it as "skin-out" biology, separating it thus from physiology, which is more largely concerned with events inside the skin of the individual. It is sometimes called a new science. But while the word itself is relatively new, dating only from 1870, the subject matter is essentially continuous with the old natural history. We can translate the title, then, into "the natural history of health," if that helps.

Curiously enough, we are more accustomed to think about the natural history of disease than about the natural history of health. Perhaps this is because we have easier access to the diseases and can isolate them for study. Particularly in the case of the infectious diseases, we can discover and describe the causative agent, the pathogen, study its interactions with the host, and its ways of getting from one host to another. A great many of the pathogens that cause disease in man have alternate hosts, or vectors, and the study of this sort of disease situation leads directly into matters that are of classical ecological and biological concern.

It is interesting that the study of the insect-borne diseases has contributed a great deal to the development of biological ecology. For instance, the understanding of jungle yellow fever in South America and Africa involved study of forest mosquitoes and mammals and led to considerable work on phenomena such as the vertical layering of climates within the rain forest. The importance of malaria in the warm regions of the world has led to a great deal of work on the ecology of the ponds, streams and marshes where the vector mosquitoes breed. In the case of African sleeping-sickness, it has turned out that the distribution of the disease partly depends on vegetation favorable to the tsetse flies, and this of course means that ecological studies of a classical sort must be made.

Our preoccupation with the ecology of disease, especially of infectious disease, is thus easy to understand. Even the purely human contagions, like measles or smallpox, depend for their maintenance and spread on factors that are familiar to the ecologists, e.g., population densities, population movement, climatic conditions, and the like. All infectious diseases involve parasitic relationships, a subject familiar enough to biologists.

The concept of disease covers a great many things beside infections—mental diseases, hereditary diseases, diseases caused by dietary deficiencies. The ecological element in some of these disease situations is slight—their understanding may depend more on such other segments of biology as genetics, physiology, or psychology—but we still somehow have the feeling that we are dealing with areas of science where entities are relatively easy to define and where classical methods of study can be used.

The ecology of health is something else. We have somehow shifted, and find ourselves looking at the landscape from a new and different point of view. "New," to be sure, is a dangerous and misleading word. As Dr. Galdston has shown, in turning our attention to health rather than to disease, we are really going back to one of the oldest traditions in medicine—going back, as we so often do, to the Greeks, to a theme in the Hippocratic writings. In modern times many critics have said that medicine is too preoccupied with disease, that it should pay more attention to the "normal state," to health. In recent years, there has undoubtedly been an increasing emphasis on this positive value of promoting health.

But what do we mean by "health"? It seems to be a very difficult concept to define with any precision. We sometimes tend to think of it in a rather negative sort of way as the absence of disease. But there are clearly degrees of health beyond the mere absence of demonstrable disease. The word carries, in fact, connotations of the "optimum," of "the best," and optimal states are notoriously difficult to define, because the optimum is meaningless except in relation to some end. In the case of health, for instance, the optimal conditions might be somewhat different depending on whether the end was maximum length of life, maximum happiness or maximum productivity. There may also, as we shall see, be some difference depending on whether we are concerned with the health of the individual, of a community, or of mankind as a whole.

Health clearly is what the students of semantics call a polar word—its meaning is relative to some standard or scale. I rather like the idea proposed by J. E. Perkins and developed by John Gordon, that "so long as life exists, some degree of health persists." The absolute zero of health, then, would be death, and there would be no fixed upper limit for the potentialities of human functioning.

We are talking, of course, about human health. Quite rightly we are being anthropocentric and not taking some cosmic point of view by which man is reduced to proper insignificance as a transient affliction of that odd little planet, Earth. But our title is general, and it may be interesting to take, for a moment, a general ecological point of view.

We are apt to think of health as the normal, natural

state of things and of disease as some departure from this norm. Yet, ecologically, it seems to me that the upper ranges of health, the sort of thing we are striving for with man, are clearly unnatural. Disease, as an aspect of parasitism, seems to be perfectly "natural." The whole system of nature is geared to a complex set of checks and balances, whereby the different populations live at the expense of each other in various sorts of food relationships—including parasitic relationships.

Malthus long ago stated the problem in his famous propositions, which have so aptly come to be called his "dismal theorem." All organisms tend to reproduce at a rate which exceeds possibility of support. Man, it seemed to Malthus, behaved like other organisms, and tended to reproduce up to the limit of his means of subsistence, which led inevitably to famine, war, disease, all the things that he lumped as the "positive check of vice and misery." Potential reproduction, we would say now, is checked by environmental resistance. Vice and misery are clearly unhealthy by any definition; but this "environmental resistance" of our modern jargon, when man encounters it, is also unhealthy.

In the biotic community, man is achieving his increasing health at the expense of the health of other organisms. Greater health for man means less health for the smallpox virus or the malaria parasite. I don't suppose that anyone is going to organize a society for the prevention of cruelty to parasites—though many people have seriously maintained that the control of infectious disease was futile or even bad because it would lead to even more serious health conditions like famine.

The fallacy here, I think, lies in regarding man as inevitably chained by the checks and balances of the natural system. I suppose we might call this the ecological fallacy, though it would perhaps more appropriately be called the ecological dilemma. The dilemma arises from the fact that man is, clearly and inevitably, a part of nature, and yet, at the same time, a most unnatural phenomenon. Man's uniqueness stems from his development of culture. It is easy to find analogues of culture, traces of culture-like phenomena, among other animals—behavior modified by learning, and transmitted from generation to generation by a sort of teaching process—but with man, these cultural modifications of behavior become so overwhelmingly important as to make the human animal a new kind of thing in nature, an "emergent." This is why biological ecology simply cannot be extended to include one more species, *Homo sapiens*; when, as human ecology, it becomes concerned primarily with human activities, it becomes a new, and in many ways, a very different science.

The lectures in this series on medicine and anthropology are mostly concerned with the relations between culture and problems of health, and I am trying to give a biological perspective to this, rather than to talk about cultural aspects of human behavior directly. But it is impossible to discuss any aspect of human behavior without taking culture into account.

Now this human culture is in itself a natural phenomenon, in the sense that we believe it started in some natural way with man's prehuman ancestors, developing in accordance with natural laws. Culture is natural in the sense that there seems to be no need to fall back on supernatural intervention to explain its development. But cultural evolution, once it started, began to operate on a quite different basis from biological evolution. The transmission of cultural traits depended, not on the continuity of the germ plasm, but on the continuity of tradition. It was based, not in genes and chromosomes, but in the development of symbolic language. This difference, among other things, led to a quite different rate of change in biological and cultural phenomena. To the extent that cultural traits differ, in their genesis, transmission and mode of change, from biological traits, they are unnatural—in the sense that they are purely and characteristically human. Man is a part of nature in that we cannot regard his activities as consequences of any special supernatural suspension of natural laws; but he is apart from nature, to the extent that his activities as a bearer of culture are peculiar. The ecological dilemma, then, is that man is both natural and unnatural, depending on the meaning given to "natural"; the ecological fallacy consists in ignoring this basic divergence.

The relationship between biological and cultural evolution presents many interesting problems that we are only beginning to understand. Some students believe that biological evolution has been suspended by the operation of cultural evolution. Some consider that culture is operating to man's biological detriment—specifically that medicine, by suspending the operation of the natural selection that would eliminate the physically defective, is endangering man's biological inheritance, and that this must be corrected by a program of artificial selection, of eugenics. My feeling is that we simply don't know enough about the operation of biological or cultural laws for intelligent decision; that whatever the biological consequences, we are caught in the stream of culture, and that we must try to operate with the currents of that stream. The problems are both urgent and fascinating. That their understanding will require the fusion of biological, medical and cultural points of view, certainly does nothing to detract from their fascination.

That health is unnatural in terms of biological ecology, then, does not bother me at all. All of medicine, all of science, is unnatural, in that it is a product of this human culture. I suppose we might use "artificial" as opposed to "natural" in this sense. But man is committed to his artifices, and there is no use in yearning after the natural health of the early Stone Age.

The problem of the meaning of health in the system of nature is partly a problem of categories. The connotations of health inevitably involve us in the concept of the optimum, and the optimum immediately raises the question of "best for what?" About the only clear answer we find in nature is "for survival and reproduction." The complex adjustments of the natural system appear to be adapted, primarily, to insure the continuity of the life process itself. The good of the species is subordinate to this. Different species, different kinds of life, may arise, flourish, and become extinct—but they are giving way to new forms, to better adapted forms, and the life process thus continues. The individual, in this grand scheme, seems to mean nothing at all. Each individual is a bundle of adaptations for survival and reproduction but, as nature is arranged, most individuals must die before they can reproduce. Life for rabbits would rapidly become impossible if all rabbits survived to reproduce, rabbit reproduction being what it is. The majority of individuals are thus doomed to an early death that the species itself can survive.

When we move from biological ecology to human ecology we change perspective, but I think it is well still to ponder the meaning of health in relation to categories. We are now dealing with one species, but we still have many groupings: the individual, the family, the community—village, city or nation—and mankind as a whole. Perhaps the same hierarchy of values should apply here; but it seems to me that the genius of man is, or could be, his concern with the individual. The ants solved the problem of community living with the individual completely subordinate many millions of years ago. Our problem is to find ways of maintaining the species and the community without sacrificing the individual. Our optimum, I think, our highest value, would be to find ways in which the meanings of health for the individual, for the nation, and for mankind as a whole, could be made to coincide.

It is not an easy problem to solve, because the interests of the individual often seem to be at variance with those of the community, and the interests of the community at variance with those of mankind as a whole. I still remember vividly a morning when I sat in on a staff meeting of the governing officials of a Pacific island. An inter-island trading ship had changed its course to drop us there the day before. The ship had then spent the night in port, but it developed that the health authorities had not allowed the crew or any of the numerous deck passengers ashore. The chief justice of the island, at the staff meeting, was quite irritated at the chief health officer. "How," he said, "can we try to instruct these people in democracy, and then, when a ship comes in, follow the undemocratic practice of allowing the American scientists and the ship's officers ashore, and preventing anyone else from landing?" But the health officer was sure of his ground. "I have finally," he said, "completely eradicated venereal disease on this island. How can I endanger this whole program, endanger the welfare of this community, by permitting almost certain contamination?"

Health and democracy, health and freedom of the individual, were clearly here in opposition. The matter was not settled at the staff meeting. I don't know that there is any rule of thumb by which conflict between individual interest and community interest can be settled. If there is a rule of thumb, I am sure it is not that the individual must be sacrificed to the community. That may be the way of nature, but I do not see why it should necessarily be the way of man. On the other hand, it is equally clear that the rule of thumb cannot be that the interests of the community must be sacrificed to those of the individual, whatever the status of the individual. That way lies chaos and ultimate misery for all.

The Pacific island incident was perhaps particularly pointed for me because it occurred against a background of an earlier discussion of "colonial" public health practices. In that earlier case, the critic of colonialism had remarked that "the ideal of you public health people would be to have the whole population in jail; then you could be sure that they had the right diet, got the right shots at the right time, were properly isolated when contagious, and all the rest."

This thought, that the ideal would be to have the whole population under complete control, sometimes seems frighteningly close to the mark. It is particularly apparent when the preoccupation is with physical health, and when health is dealt with as a sort of commodity in intercultural contacts. It is the logic of totalitarianism, of the "Brave New World" that sometimes seems to be taking shape under our very noses.

We have, however, in many places and at various times achieved what seem to be reasonable solutions to the problems of conflict of interest between the health of the individual and the health of the community. The problems here seem almost trivial when compared with the problems of conflict of interest between the health of the community and the health of mankind as a whole. To realize the gravity of the problem, we have only, in contemporary times, to concentrate on a particular kind of community, the national state, and look at the apparent discrepancies between the health of a particular state and the health of the human species, whether as a whole or as an agglomeration of individuals—everyone of them terribly and rightfully important to himself.

I was reading the other day a description of the health of the armed forces of a particular nation. It was a glowing account of success—I was reminded again of the point about jails made by my anti-colonial friend. If you can't get the whole population in jail, the next best thing is to get as large a part of it as possible into the army. There, you can not only look after their physical health, but you can tinker, sometimes successfully, with their psychology, their morale, their education. The armed forces of every modern state are splendid examples of what can be accomplished through the application of health techniques. Hans Zinsser, in his delightful book on *Rats, Lice and History,* has a chapter on the "Unimportance of Generals" in which he makes the point that more wars have been decided by pathogens than by military strategy (4). Historically, this seems quite probable; but the pathogens have been licked and the generals are now assured of a ready supply of healthy cannon fodder.

But what a queer contradiction of terms this is, the "health of the armed forces"; the maintenance of health for the furtherance of the worst disease of all, war.

I do not think I have strayed from my topic, the ecology of health in man. Health is life; its complete absence is death. War and health are completely contradictory.

Let us look for a moment at that absolute zero of health, death. We can classify the causes of death in many different ways. A basic division that can be made is between physiological death and ecological death: death from the running down of the time-clock that seems to be built into every organism, or from defects inherent in the organism; and death brought about by agencies external to the organism. If we try, further, to classify different forms of ecological death, we come up with categories like parasitism, predation, starvation, and accidents or various sorts of hazards of the physical environment.

When we try to survey the ecological causes of death in man, however, we find, in addition to the general categories that seem to apply to all sorts of organisms, a special category, that of men killing each other. This phenomenon is common and ubiquitous in man, and it goes back as far as we can peer into human history and prehistory. But it seems to be uniquely human, and I have difficulty finding analogues or precedents among any other kinds of organisms. Certainly many animals kill and eat each other in confinement, and overcrowding may sometimes lead to such behavior in nature, though it is hard to get evidence. Some invertebrates seem to rely on the young eating each other as a way of getting a start in life—a sort of alternative to providing extra yolk. The female spiders and mantis that eat their mates are notorious—but the male is generally eaten after the female has been fertilized, when he is no longer of any use. And of course the males of many animals fight among themselves to gain possession of females, but cases in which such combat is fatal are extremely rare.

The usual analogies between warlike behavior and predatory behavior are inapplicable, because predation involves one kind of animal, one species, killing and eating some other kind of animal. This is true also of the well-publicized wars, slave-raids and the like among ants. Man killing man is an example of individuals of a given species regularly and systematically killing other members of the same species. This indeed is "unnatural."

The only good biological analogy I can find is that of behavior associated with territoriality in mammals and other vertebrates. "Territory" in ecology is defined as an area defended against members of the same species. The territory may be staked out and defended by individual males, by families, or by superfamilial, tribe-like groups, as in monkeys and wolves. I do not know of any case, however, where territorial squabbling in nature leads directly to the death of any of the individuals concerned, though it may be an indirect cause of death, since individuals unable to establish or preempt territories frequently become the victims of predation.

All of the primates that have been studied in the field show territorial behavior, and we can be quite sure that man's prehuman ancestors were territorial, as are the living primates. Konrad Lorenz has suggested that in the biological evolution of behavior, the development of weapons like teeth or claws that might enable one individual to kill another of the same species has always been accompanied by the evolution of inhibiting behavior to prevent such intraspecific killing. If human warfare has its biological origins in this territorial behavior, its lethal nature may perhaps be explained by a failure in cultural evolution—as stones and clubs developed into bows and spears and rifles and cannon, the corresponding development of cultural inhibitions failed to take place. I find this a comforting theory because cultural change can occur with great rapidity as compared with biological change. If culture can produce the armaments, surely it can produce the inhibitions. The realization that the inhibitions are absolutely necessary for the survival of the species may provide the incentive. At least I see no other way out of the box we are in.

The ancientness of this cultural practice of men killing each other is curious. Franz Weidenreich, who was a physician as well as an anthropologist, undertook a study of the duration of life of fossil man in China. It turned out to be quite easy to establish the primary cause of death for these fossils. In every case there was evidence that the man had been killed by some other man. This was true of the very old fossils of Pekin Man, the Sinanthropus of the Choukoutien Cave. All of the long bones found in this cave had been split open: which anthropologists take as direct evidence of cannibalism, since only a fellow man would split open a bone to get at the marrow. The skulls also all showed evidence of heavy blows. Thus, way back in the early Stone Age, it appears that murder, with cannibal intent, was a well-established human practice.

The late Stone Age fossils examined by Weidenreich also showed evidence that men killed each other. One skull, he wrote, "shows a long and wide slit-like hole at the superior part of the left temporal region . . . giving the impression that it was caused by a spear-like implement piercing through the wall from above" (3).

What is the explanation of the development of this peculiar human behavior? If it evolved from territorial squabbling, it may be related to population growth. It seems clear that territorial behavior in mammals, birds and the like, serves a function of spacing the population. The territory staked out by a given pair of nesting songbirds, for instance, appears to include populations of insects and other good eatables rather in excess of the needs of the territory owners. To go back to that dismal theorem of Malthus, that populations tend to live up to the means of subsistence, it appears that this must be modified, even in terms of biological ecology, in that there are checks interposed on populations which tend to prevent their growth up to this ultimate limit of the means of subsistence. This must be so, because a population living up to the limit of its food supply would be liable, at any moment, to catastrophe; and nature seems generally to be a smoothly running affair, with catastrophes—where man has not interfered—notably rare. I don't want to go into the general problem of checks on populations in nature—if for no other reason than the very good one that I don't understand them—but it looks as though availability of territory were one such check.

It appears that with many mammals and birds, the individuals that cannot establish territories fail to reproduce, and that such individuals are particularly likely to fall victim to passing predators—hawks, foxes, lions or what have you. By way of aside, I have long wanted to know what, in nature, controls the lion population. When left alone, apparently they do not live up to the limit of the supply of gazelles, otherwise the last gazelle would long since have disappeared down some lion gullet. But no one so far has been able to answer my lion question!

With Stone Age man, it seems possible that territorial squabbling, when cultural evolution reached the point where the territorial intruder was directly killed, there was a further development of territory functioning as a check on population.

Of course, there are several long leaps between territoriality in primates, evidence of murder in early man, territoriality and primitive warfare among contemporary food-gathering peoples, and that phenomenon we call modern war. Food-gathering man, I suspect, showed territorial behavior not too unlike that shown by our living primates. But this pattern disappeared with the cultural changes involved in the shift from food-gathering to food-producing, with the aggregation of people into villages and presently into cities and towns. When we get to agricultural tribes, to cities, empires and nations, we have phenomena that have no counterparts with other organisms. We have learned to be very dubious about the attribution of "instincts" to man, and it is hard to believe that some vague sort of biological territorial instinct would carry over to account for the continuation of conflict among these various sorts of social organizations. But perhaps it was the cultural habit of man killing man that carried over, taking new forms as new forms of social organization were developed. Whatever the genesis, we are faced with the fact that man is still killing man, and that this is a major ecological hazard to his health, whether as an individual, a community, or a species.

This human habit is so peculiar from a biological point of view that it seems to me that it ought to have a special name. Terms like "suicide" and "homicide" which first come to mind can hardly be used because they already have definite and restricted meanings. I became preoccupied with this while writing a recent book and I asked a friend who was also a Greek scholar what could be done with a Greek root. He suggested "anthropoktony" from *anthropos,* man, and *ktonos,* to kill. Ecology, as a science, is notable for its jargon. Any ecologist can take a simple idea and make it unintelligible by dressing it up with big words. My favorite definition of ecology is one I learned from Karl Schmidt—"that science in which a spade is called a geotome." So I have no qualms about adding to the jargon. And anthropoktony seems a fittingly horrible word for the curious biological perversion to which it refers.

Anthropoktony takes endlessly diverse forms, and I think it would have to figure largely in any ecological study of human health. People kill each other for private reasons and for public reasons, with the sanction of society and without it. They even deliberately and consciously kill themselves, finding life intolerable. All of these forms of anthropoktony present problems in relation to the ecology of health, even though they are mostly trivial when compared with that great health problem of our time, modern war.

There is a theory that modern war is a consequence of the so-called "population problem." I am concerned enough about the rate of growth of human population and about the continuation of war and the threat of war, but I have never been able to see the direct relation between the two in modern times. The effect of constant, attritional warfare among many primitive peoples is easy to see, and such warfare, through much of human prehistory, may have been the actual check on population growth. A classic case would be that in which a man must get the head of an enemy to prove his manhood before he can settle down with a wife and start a family. Such systems serve obviously enough as checks on population growth.

But the most rapid growth of human populations has taken place in modern times, when wars have been prevalent enough and devastating enough; clearly they are not a practical check on population growth. I fail to see any connection betwen density of population and warlikeness —some of the most crowded parts of the world are also among the most peaceful. The Hitlerian shout of need for *Lebensraum* while urging the German people to breed ever more recklessly is proof enough of the absurdity of the argument. More and more it seems to me true that wars begin in the minds of men—and it is through the minds of men that we must find the cure.

Though I would regard war and population as separate problems in the ecology of human health, and consider war to be the most urgent of all human problems, population seems hardly less important. Again we are dealing with a product of cultural evolution rather than biological evolution. All through nature there is a rather close adjustment between the reproduction rate of a given species and the hazards of its existence, so that the elephant birth rate is in accord with the hazards of elephant existence and the oyster birth rate in accord with oyster hazards. The hazards of human existence have changed rapidly in modern times through cultural developments like medicine, public health and technology, and it sometimes looks as though this has become dangerously out of phase with changes in the reproduction rate.

Actually, within the culture that we call Western Civilization, we can see that the downward trends in mortality rates have been roughly paralleled by downward trends in birth rates, though sometimes with considerable lag. Cultural evolution seems to be operating in much the same way as biological evolution. This is curious because the mortality rates have changed, in part at least, as a result of deliberate and planned intervention through medicine and public health. Medical developments have certainly also been influential in lowering the birth rates—but without benefit of planned, governmental organization of either research or application.

The situation is different, however, in terms of cross-cultural relations in connection with technological development. Modern medical techniques, with governmental backing, can bring about swift changes in the mortality pattern of a population corresponding to changes that have occurred rather slowly in the West, where there was time for various sorts of cultural adjustment. Can the non-Western countries of the world afford to make this swift change in mortality without giving equally conscious attention to patterns of reproduction? The problem certainly worries leaders in Japan and India. But it is a problem shared by the whole world-community and we ought to cooperate in studying it.

The technologists seem very confident that the world can easily support a very much larger number of humans than are presently living on it. We can use nuclear energy, and live on algae soup, perhaps breeding to the ultimate of standing room only. I am willing to believe them. The problem of the numbers of men seems to be not so much resources as organization. Harrison Brown has made this point clearly in his book, *The Challenge of Man's Future* (1). With tight organization—totalitarian organization—the resources of the world can be manipulated, populations controlled, people crowded together indefinitely as long as they are well policed. We approach the ideal of Huxley's *Brave New World* (2) of having the whole population in jail.

Health is concerned not only with the welfare of man's body, but also with the welfare of his mind and soul. Even if we can provide for man's body, can we provide for his mind and soul in an overcrowded world? There are signs already that we are failing here. No one will dispute our progress in controlling the ills of the body, in promoting physical health. We are far from any ideal, but the dead weight of pain, illness and physical misery is demonstrably less from year to year.

It is difficult to say as much for men's minds and souls. Of course, hard as it is to set a goal for man's physical health, it is far harder to define a goal for mental health. We are faced again with the problem of defining the optimum, and the optimum will vary in terms of the values used for measuring it.

Surely, however, there is a relation between physical health and mental health. In reducing the sheer volume of physical misery in the world, I suspect that we have also reduced the mental misery. But I doubt whether there would be universal agreement with this—and I think some would maintain that we have become sicker in mind as we have become healthier in body. A case certainly can be made out, with statistics on increases in psychoses, in crime, in delinquency, in various sorts of social ills. For an over-all appraisal, we should have to decide somehow whether the deviant cases, the victims of our progress, outweigh the mass who have gained in security, in enjoyed leisure, in happiness. I think that so far we have gained rather than lost; but statistics on happiness are hard to come by, and I am unable to prove my point.

I do think, however, that the danger is very real. Man's destiny is not to repeat the social experiment of the ants. He is not built that way. But a respectable portion of the world's population seems already committed to an ant-like integration of the individual into society. This, to be sure, is supposed to be a temporary phase, with government presently withering away to leave men free. I am no expert in the natural history of governments, but it seems to me hardly likely that any government will ever wither away unless someone has previously used an axe on it. In fact, the growing population of the world and the ever-increasing complexity of the technology required for the support of that population seems to demand ever more complex organization, ever stronger and more central government. The population and resource situation of the world today makes competing nationalisms anachronistic, makes the need for continuing the development of forms of world organization imperative. This appears to be a consequence of the course of cultural evolution, inevitable whether we like it or not—unless, of course, we stop cultural evolution by blowing ourselves up.

I think I have not strayed from my topic of the ecology of health; rather I have stopped to glance at some of the great issues of health, those that concern the welfare of mankind as a whole.

But what happens to the individual? How, in the face of the growing complexity of the human situation, can he maintain—or increase—his individuality, his freedom and integrity? I firmly believe that the greatness of man turns on these values, that our destiny lies in cultivating them. But this is not easy. The needs of the state and of mankind often seem to transcend those of the individual. Fundamentally, the health of mankind and the health of the state depend on the health of individuals—their health in mind and soul as well as in body—but this fundamental unity is overlaid by a chaos of diversity and apparent conflict of interest. To find this unity, explain it, and implement it, this is the great problem of the ecology of health.

REFERENCES

1. Brown, Harrison: *The Challenge of Man's Future.* New York: Viking Press, 1956.
2. Huxley, Aldous: *Brave New World.* New York: Harper, 1932.
3. Weidenreich, Franz: The Duration of Life of Fossil Man in China and the Pathological Lesions Found in His Skeleton. *Chinese Medical Journal, 55*:34-44, 1939. Reprinted in *Anthropological Papers of Franz Weidenreich.* New York: The Viking Fund, 1949.
4. Zinsser, Hans: *Rats, Lice and History.* Boston: Little, Brown, 1935.

CULTURAL MENTALITIES AND MEDICAL SCIENCE

By F. S. C. Northrop, Ph.D.

ONE OF THE major developments of this century is the insight into the diversity of human mentalities which has come from cultural anthropology and the comparative philosophy of the world's cultures. This insight is already transforming the lawyer's conception of law, the militarist's plans concerning strategy and the statesman's awareness of what he and his diplomats must know if foreign policy is to be based on objective knowledge of what other people think and are most likely to do rather than upon wishful thinking. The implications for medicine are equally important.

These implications show in three major ways: (1) When modern Western medical practices are applied to non-Western people; (2) when people with one cultural mentality migrate to a nation or area whose people have a different cultural mentality; (3) when diseases, prevalent and often incurable in modern Western societies, are not found among so-called primitive people.

APPLICATION OF WESTERN MEDICAL SCIENCE TO NON-WESTERN PEOPLES

Any traveler to the Far East, the Middle East, Africa or even across the Rio Grande into Mexico knows what it means to have dysentery. He soon learns that he must avoid uncooked vegetables and drink only boiled water. Even these precautions turn out, as a rule, to be insufficient. In fact prolonged living in some of these countries, even when the Western housewife continuously supervises the native cook, carries with it frequent bouts of intestinal disturbances. Nor do lectures to the native cook or even the native public health officers about "night soil" and polluted water suffice to remove the disease. A few examples from the writer's personal experience will make this clear.

In 1949 the writer was in Mexico City conversing with Dr. Manuel Gamio, the Director of the Instituto Indigenista Interamericano. Dr. Gamio described the failure of an attempt made by Mexican public health officers to purify the water supply of a local Indian village by the simple and normally sufficient procedure of adding certain chemicals at specified intervals. Not only did all efforts to this end fail, but a bitter reaction of the natives resulted. Investigation of the source of the bitterness revealed that in their conception of natural phenomena, water was regarded not merely as the creative source of human life but also as the model of goodness and even of the sacred. Thus in the native mind, to put chemicals in the local water supply was to tamper with the morally good and to be guilty of sacrilege. From the standpoint of their mentality, the water supply in its natural state was good; for it to be bad, in a medical or in any other way, was to them unthinkable. In classical Chinese thinking, also, water is regarded as the model for human conduct since by its resiliency it is never destroyed when struck with the hardest object and is able with time to wear away mountains.

This example suffices to make one principle clear. Effective medical science must give as much attention to the cultural mentality of the patient as to the chemistry of his disease.

In 1950 the writer was taken by an American doctor through the native village of a country bordering on the Mediterranean. The capital of this nation has been under dominant modern Western influence for centuries. The doctor, who represented the medical division of one of America's major foundations, was supervising the public health program of the native village. This village, but sixty miles from the capital city, had been chosen for an experimental health program because its health conditions were found, after an international survey, to be about the worst in the world. Within a period of three years Western doctors working with native assistants had succeeded, by relatively simple and inexpensive procedures, in raising the health of this village practically to the level of modern Western society. However, as we drove back to the capital, the American doctor said that the prospects were not too encouraging because previous experience had shown that when the Western medical supervisors leave, the health conditions tend to return to their previous state, notwithstanding the native health officer's continued use of the modern Western ways.

In support of this judgment the American doctor described the following experience. Some ten years before, in another village in the same nation, Western doctors had not merely raised the health of the village approximately to modern Western standards, but were also convinced that they had trained a native public health officer in the knowledge of what to do to keep it there and in grasping the Western scientific mentality necessary to understand why it had to be done that way. Nevertheless, with the departure of the Western advisors the health of the village reverted approximately to its original low state. The new practices were continued in a mechanical way but with old social habits accompanying them and with corners cut here and there in such a manner that the pollutions and infections returned. It became evident that the native health officer, for all his modern indoctrination and practices, did not understand what he was doing.

Dr. Lyle Saunders describes similar behavior on the part of the Spanish Mexicans in the southwestern United States. Not only are the old medical ways preferred, but:

> if the Anglo methods are adopted, their efficacy may be reduced by the failure . . . to grasp the reasons behind their use. The scissors, after being washed with soap, may be dried with an unsterile cloth or placed on a table that has not been cleaned. Water that has been boiled may be poured when cool into an unsterile container . . . the new procedures are not understood in terms of the Anglo reasons for their use, but instead are fitted into the already existing pattern of understanding with respect to causation and healing of illness and disease (7, p. 158).

The reference to "causation" is important, since it shows that even a primitive people have a particular philosophy of natural science.

These experiences make another principle clear. Effective medical science is more than a set of concrete practical prescriptions for the cure of specific unhealthy conditions; it is also a comprehensive way of thinking about every fact of nature and every act of daily life upon the part of the physician, the public health officer and the patients. Practical prescriptions without the philosophy of natural science, which they presuppose for their meaningfulness, and without the philosophy of social behavior and of culture, which they need for their reinforcement, are frequently worthless.

A fourth concrete experience will indicate why this is the case. The occasion was January, 1953, in the office of the Ambassador of the United States in a South American country. The Ambassador spoke of the experiences of a medical commission which had been investigating the malnutrition of Indians in that country's High Andes. The investigations had shown that it seemed unwise for the United States to appropriate Truman Point Four Aid to increase the productivity of the native Indian agriculture before certain medical programs were introduced. The reason was that the Indians, due to a chronic intestinal infection, were able to derive from their existent food supply only forty per cent of its normal nutriment. Hence, the eradication of this infection by drugs, which is relatively easy chemically, would be equivalent to more than doubling the food supply. Unfortunately, this medical program failed for the simple reason that the natives' daily habits of walking barefoot and sleeping on earthen floors produced reinfections faster than the drugs could cure them.

This experience shows that the effectiveness of a drug in destroying the bacterial infection of a people depends not merely on the demonstrated chemical capacity of the drug to kill that bacterium when isolated in a pharmacologist's laboratory, but also on the waking and sleeping habits of the people to whom the drug is given, which in turn derive from the people's mentality. Without altering the way in which they think about the earth and water supply and what each contains by way of entities dangerous to health, and about the relation of their bare feet or their washed vegetables to earth and water—i.e., without altering their basic philosophy of natural phenomena, so that in every moment of their waking, and perhaps even their sleeping, lives they clothe themselves and behave in a new way—the modern drug may be of little avail.

The foregoing considerations do not mean that there is no effective way to apply modern Western medicine to non-Western people. They do mean, however, that for success to ensue, both the scientific and cultural mentality behind modern Western medical ways and the different mentality of the native people must be taken into account and combined so that the one reinforces the other. In other words, effective medical science is concerned with the relation between a specific set of practical prescriptions and two different mentalities: (1) The mentality specified by the basic concepts or philosophy of the physical, physiological, chemical and psychological sciences, which must be grasped if the cause of the disease and the accompanying personal and social practices necessary for its medical cure are to be known and understood, and (2) the mentality specified by the way of thinking about natural phenomena and personal and social behavior, i.e., the philosophy of nature and of culture of the patient or the people to whom the medical prescriptions are given. As Dr. Lyle Saunders, generalizing from his medical experience with the Spanish-speaking people of the southwestern United States, has written in his book, *Cultural Difference and Medical Care*:

> the practice of medicine always involves interaction between two or more socially conditioned human beings [and] . . . takes place within a social system that defines the roles of the participants, specifies the kinds of behavior appropriate to each of those roles, and provides the sets of values in terms of which the participants are motivated (7, p. 7).

When (a) the medical prescriptions and public health practices and (b) the basic scientific and cultural mentality which they presuppose for their effectiveness are those of the culture of the patient, as is the case with patients born and educated in modern Western cultures, the mentality of the patient tends automatically to provide the state of mind and the daily behavior necessary to make the medical practice effective. In the United States, for example, the people generally have become so accustomed to thinking about themselves and the phenomena of nature in terms of unobservable or exceedingly microscopic entities, such as atoms, electrons and bacteria, that the conception of clear water as polluted or the danger of eating vegetables fertilized by human excrement, presents little if any problem for them.

It does not follow, however, that the diversity of cultural mentalities generates no problems for medical science in modern Western societies. There are immigrants in the United States.

MEDICAL PROBLEMS THAT ARISE WHEN PEOPLE MIGRATE TO A NATION WITH A DIFFERENT CULTURAL MENTALITY

The Puerto Rican community in New York City provides one example, the early Italian community in New Haven another. There are, of course, many more examples in other nations as well as in the United States. Most of the Puerto Ricans in New York or the Italians in New Haven come from peasant communities. These peasant communities have their indigenous norms and standards which give each person his or her emotional sense of belonging and the moral rules for social conduct. Hence, as the sequel will show, most of these immigrants in the United States were, in the land of their birth, reasonably at peace with themselves emotionally and morally responsible socially.

Consider what happens to these first generation Puerto Rican and Italian immigrants when they place their children in the public schools of New York City and New Haven. To begin with, English rather than Spanish or Italian is the required language. Moreover, it must be spoken, if the sensitive child is not to be teased and made miserable by his or her fellow students, with an American rather than a Spanish or Italian accent (1, pp. 21-24, 79-82; 9, pp. 131-134). This American-English the boys and girls soon acquire at school. But struggle as they may, it is too much for their parents at home on 120th Street or East Grand Avenue—the Spanish or Italian accent persists. In the child's mind, however, as fashioned in school, to speak broken English is not to belong; it is to be not truly American (1, pp. 101-105). Under such circumstances it is very difficult, if not impossible, for the first generation boys and girls to avoid being emotionally disturbed by, if not socially ashamed of, the speech of their parents. Here arises the first break between the parents and their children.

Nor does the curriculum of the school help matters. It is Anglo-American literature and Anglo-American legally constructed and individualistically centered social theory, not Italian or Spanish literature or Italian and Puerto Rican emotionally felt and family-centered social behavior which are taught. Also, above everything else, civics and the American way of life must be emphasized (1, p. 40 ff; 9, pp. 133-134). Certainly, it will be said, this is all to the good. Do not the Declaration of Independence and the Constitution of the United States with its Bill of Rights give these new Americans both the opportunity and the protection of their liberty to believe and to worship as they deem best? The answer, of course, is "Yes." But in doing these things, which are obviously good from the standpoint of the Puerto Rican and Italian immigrants as well as the rest of us, this same American constitution does one other thing which those of us who cherish its many merits have overlooked. It means, to use the language of Sir Henry S. Maine in his classic work, *Ancient Law,* that these children of newly arrived Italian and Puerto Rican parents are being shifted from the family-centered and -supervised personal and social ethics of the law of status mentality of their parents to the legally constructed and contracted, individualistically centered personal and social ethics of the law of contract mentality of the new community. Forthwith, not only do the Italian or Puerto Rican parents fail to speak the same language as their children but they also find themselves and their children meaning different things by the word "good" when any language is spoken.

It may also be said that neither the parents nor the children know anything about the distinctions between the law of status and the law of contract. This, unfortunately, is true and makes matters all the worse, for neither party understands what is happening. Both the newly arrived parents and the first generation children do know very well, however, that in the United States it is proper for young boys and girls to sit together in the same classroom, to make public social engagements wholly independently, without consulting their families, and to carry out those public engagements without the continuous observation and chaperonage of their own parents or any other parents. This means concretely that the individual young person is being related to the sanction for moral and legal behavior not mediately, by way of his parents and family, as the law of status society requires, but directly, by his or her own independent decision and consent to contractually constructed legal statutes or social engagements, after the manner of the law of contract.

To see why this gives rise to serious medical, social, legal and moral problems for both the parents and the children, it is necessary to examine the mentality and social ways of the cultures from which the parents have emigrated. Such an examination has been carried through by Phyllis H. Williams (9) for the south Italian villages from which "the great majority of Italian immigrants in New Haven" (1, p. 20) have come. Her study shows the following things.

First the communities are village communities dominated by the *campanilismo* mentality (9, p. 34). *Campanilismo* means "that which is within sound of the village bell" (9, p. 9). This mentality expresses the fact that for these people "the commune [or village] is everything and the State is very little" (9, p. 8). In other words, the widest acceptable social norms are those between the villagers, practically all of whom know one another. For example, in one of the states in southern Italy there are ninety-one villages which have practically no connection with one another and accept little if any political authority beyond the local village (9, p. 9). As one New Haven Italian who had just returned from a visit to the land of his birth said: "I say (sic) Italy; but for me, as for the others, Italy is the little village where I was raised" (9, p. 17).

Secondly, these southern Italians do not speak the Italian of Rome and the northern cities; each village or local area speaks its own dialect. This generates the *paesano* mentality. *Paesano* means "a person from the same [linguistic] district or town as the speaker" (9, pp. 10-11, 46). This mentality has important moral and social consequences. First, it is regarded as bad for a child of one village or local linguistic district to marry the child of another. Second, hospitals are bad and are to be avoided, as are doctors from Naples, Rome or northern Italy who are trained in modern Western ways. The reason for this moral judgment is that these hospitals and doctors are introduced and financed in considerable part by the federal government and the *campanilismo-paesano* mentality causes anything coming from outside the village to be regarded as bad. The villagers believe also in a different type of medical practice which, as Williams (9, pp. 160-182) and Sigerist have shown, is typical of so-called primitive people the world over (8, pp. 121, 209). This belief leads them to regard hospitals merely as devices of the doctors to make use of the native villagers as experimental material for the study of diseases which the doctors do not know how to cure. Needless to say, this mentality has produced problems for the medical profession and the visiting nurses when these villagers have emigrated to New Haven, Connecticut (9, pp. 174-182).

Another characteristic of the southern Italian native mentality is an "inclination to procrastinate" (9, p. 8) and a "take it easy" attitude (9, p. 33). This way of thinking and behaving is called *pazienza. Pazienza* means patience. *Pazienza* leads modern westerners, probably somewhat erroneously, to describe primitive people as "fatalistic" (9, p. 8). *Pazienza* is more correctly described as behavior in accord with the immediately felt and sensed rhythms of nature in which one is immersed. This attitude is not peculiar to southern Italy. As a French observer noted at the beginning of the nineteenth century, "Europe ends at Naples, and it ends there badly enough. Calabria, Sicily, all the rest is African" (9, p. 1).

This identification of the mentality of the south Italian with the African mentality, by way of contrast, means that

Naples, Rome and northern Italy have been Romanized. To be Romanized is to be brought not merely under the medical, moral and social ways of thinking of Greek mathematical science but also under the universalized personal, social and political norms, broken free from family, village and tribal ties, of the Stoic Roman lawyer's *jus gentium* and the Roman Christian Church Catholic. The universalizing mentality of the Stoic Roman lawyer's *jus gentium* (5) is the origin of Western legal science and its law of contract (2, 6). Let it not be forgotten that the literal meaning of the word "catholic" is "universal." It is this universalizing mentality of Greek mathematical physics and Stoic Roman law, passing over later into the Roman Catholic Church, which begins the lengthy process of freeing moral and social man from family, village and tribal man, to identify the moral person and the citizen instead with individualistically assenting and contractually specified universal man. This is the universalizing mentality also which went into the Declaration of Independence, the Bill of Rights and the Constitution of the United States and which expressed itself recently through the Supreme Court in its momentous decision on segregation in the schools of the United States. It is this same difference between the Italian parents' law of status family- and village-centered mentality and the law of contract mentality and its moral and social ways that gives these parents their shock when their children come home from the public schools in New Haven.

Our comprehension of the depth and magnitude of this shock will become even more evident if we shift our attention from the *campanilismo-paesano-pazienza* mentality of the southern Italian village communities from which they come to the morally proper behavior of boys and girls within these villages. The family in southern Italy is extremely patriarchal in character. This means that the father is not merely the head but also has absolute power and authority not merely to thrash his children but also to beat his wife. Moreover, such fatherly discipline is regarded as morally good by both the mother and the children (9, pp. 92-93). So much is this the case that the wife gives her husband absolute devotion and loyalty, even when he does not deserve it. The practical consequences are interesting. Both illegitimacy and abandonment of children are lower in southern Italy than in northern Italy or the United States; also "divorce was unknown" (9, p. 74).

Such patriarchal moral authority does not mean that the moral status of the mother in such families is a completely secondary or degrading one. With her children, her authority is absolute. "I obey my mother's word, which is like the God," is the way one Italian son has described her moral position (9, pp. 76-77). The mother has two other major responsibilities. She selects the wives for her sons. She is also the keeper of the family purse. Her husband's as well as her unmarried children's earnings go into this purse. Again we see the law of status ethical mentality at work. What an individual earns, even when he is the head of the family, is not his; it is the trust of the family and the mother is the executrix of that trust. Also the mate that a son chooses for his wife is not his to select; it is that of his family as arranged by his mother in negotiation with the mothers of other families solely within the village or *paesano* community. Is it surprising, therefore, when Williams finds such beliefs "color[ing] the lives of even third-generation Italians" (9, p. xv) in New Haven that she finds also that "Many Italian parents there bitterly dislike the kind of man that America makes available as a mate for their daughters" (9, p. 97).

The mother has another responsibility which is instrumental in the selection of proper wives for her sons and the securing of proper husbands for her daughters. Any morally or socially acceptable daughter must go to her wedding-bed a virgin. This is a real, not a nominal, requirement and necessitates consequently, that no morally and socially acceptable daughter can be seen in public with a young man unless accompanied by and under the direct observation of her mother. For this reason, the classrooms for boys and girls in southern Italy are in different buildings on opposite sides of the village. Even when an engagement has been arranged by the parents, the young man and the young woman can meet but three times between the date of engagement and the moment of marriage and these three meetings must be in the home of the boy's parents with the young man and the young woman continuously on different sides of the room (9, pp. 80-97).

The Indians of Mexico exhibit a similar mentality. If, in the village of Taxco, one goes on a Saturday evening to the delightfully located bar, designed for tourists, overlooking the main village square by the baroque cathedral, one will see mothers entering this square from every direction accompanied by their daughters, as the young men and their fathers enter independently. Some of the fathers, carrying musical instruments, proceed to the bandstand in the middle of the square. Around the square there is a very wide walk lined on the inner side with wooden benches. The mothers with their daughters seat themselves on these benches, while those fathers in the band prepare to play and the other men and boys form little conversational cliques around the square. When the band strikes up, the daughters arise from the benches and walk in arm-locked groups of twos and threes in one direction around the square while the young men walk in the opposite direction. After a time a young man selects a young woman and they walk around together. Shortly more and more of such pairs form. The social ceremony continues until the band plays its final piece and the daughters with their mothers return home together. The important thing about this custom is that everything occurs under the eyes of the parents and with the parents of one family conversing with those of another.

This interesting social ceremony enables us to understand and appreciate the emotional and moral disturbances that occur when such parents, living in New York or New Haven, see what happens to their children in our modern schools. Not only do they find themselves beginning to be alienated from one another because of the parents' broken English and the children's enforced and glib "Americanese," but there is also the shock to the parents of seeing the young boys and girls going off to school together with no parent of any girl continuously watching her. This is followed by the even more disturbing experience of learning that one's daughter has made a social engagement with a boy without the parents of both being consulted or being acquainted with one another. But even this experience is as nothing to the one which occurs when that girl returns home late in the evening from several hours of public or semi-public association with a boy under no parental chaperonage whatever.

To appreciate the magnitude of this emotional and moral shock, it is necessary to know the way Italians in southern Italy think about women. Every woman falls into one of two classes. The first class contains (a) those unmarried girls who never appear in public except with their mothers and (b) those married women who never appear in public except with their husband or with another married woman who is a *paesano*, i.e., a married woman who speaks the village or local dialect. Any other unmarried girl or married woman is immoral not merely in theory but also in all likelihood in fact. Moreover, the latter type of woman is regarded as morally fair game for any man. The double standard of morality for men arises precisely from the latter belief.

It will be well for modern criminal lawyers, judges and policemen, with their law of contract mentality, to keep the foregoing way of thinking about women in public and proper behavior for young men in public in mind when they come upon the deeds of passion and force of youths in our modern Western cities. To realize the cultural mentality and morality of the community from which the youths' parents and perhaps even they may have come is to see that we are confronted here with the moral confusion that must result when a woman appears in public in a way which, from the standpoint of her cultural mentality, is proper and, from the standpoint of a youth on the street with a different cultural mentality, is improper and hence in his mind is an invitation to a particular response on his part which in her culture is a crime and in his culture is morally and legally sanctioned.

Need one wonder, also, that when an Italian parent in New York or New Haven, recently arrived from southern Italy, sees his high school daughter come in at 10 o'clock at night from an unchaperoned date with a young man whom the father or mother does not know, and whose family they do not know, that

> To the girl's parents, this [behavior] portends nothing but evil. They cannot conceive of such a free social life not leading to further liberties of an indiscreet nature. . . . Some Italian parents, in fact, excited by the threat of such "wild" behavior to their family honor, have succeeded in placing their daughters in institutions for wayward girls (9, p. 98).

Need one wonder also that these immigrant parents believe that the coeducation of the American public school system has "devastated" their own morality?

The effect upon the sons and daughters of these parents is equally disturbing and demoralizing. The girl who came in at 10 o'clock knows that what she has done has been innocent and that such social behavior is regarded as quite proper by her non-Italian classmates and their parents. Yet these ways are not understood by her parents. Hence she has no way of explaining her behavior to her parents to ease their moral consternation and worst fears. Nor, if she follows her parents' moral convictions and advice by breaking off all such social engagements with her non-Italian classmates, can she make such behavior intelligible to them. Under such circumstances deep-seated emotional and neurotic conflicts are inevitable. Furthermore, Williams' investigations show that "In fighting straight-laced parental demands, recriminations follow and then beatings, and the rift [between parent and child] grows wider" (9, p. 98).

Child has made a study of the consequences. Three major types of reaction occur. One he terms the "rebel reaction." It consists in a break from the parents. The second is the "ingroup reaction." In it the son or daughter attempts to remain within the parental family and its mentality and ways. The third is the "apathetic reaction." It attempts to combine the two and results in the lack of joy and spontaneity which the adjective "apathetic" describes (1, pp. 76-187).

The ingroup reaction is probably doomed to failure by the overwhelming dominance of the larger community. In New Haven Italians are one quarter of the population. The rebel reaction leads naturally to marrying a non-Italian American. The results of this are likely to be tragic. Notwithstanding the acceptance of the new mentality, the old ways are in one emotionally and unconsciously and carry into, as noted above, the third generation. The following is an instance of what may happen. A young second generation Italian married to a non-Italian wife came into the social agency in New Haven asking for instructions on how to obtain an immediate divorce.

> He had come for dinner and washed his hands in the sink. Turning to reach for the towel, which [according to his parents' example] his wife was supposed to be holding dutifully for him, he saw her sitting in a chair reading the newspaper and paying no attention to him. He reproved her irritably, and she answered, "I am not your towel rack!" He could hardly believe his ears. Forgetting about dinner, he left immediately to find his way to the social agency [9, p. 92].

Williams notes that, "Both had sloughed off parts of the old code. After all, he too was sinning [according to his parents' code] in contemplating divorce rather than mere separation" (9, p. 92). Here we come to the real tragedy of the situation. The boy is torn away from the moral norms of his parents' mentality by the acceptance of certain ways of the new community while also being captured unconsciously and habitually by the ways of his parents. The danger then is that the child falls between both moral worlds. Torn by emotional conflicts within himself, force and the flouting of the moral rules of both communities may then seem to be the only way to affirm his integrity.

Consider also the similar plight of the Italian daughter who is unable to resist the morally accepted ways of the American school community yet having the southern Italian daughter's affection for her mother. She, too, is torn by the conflict between these ways and her mother's morality. A Sicilian lament expresses the latter tie as follows:

Take this letter to my mother,
And if she weeps, tell her that I too weep,
Thinking how strange it is that I am in this far-off land [9, p. 45].

Is it a wonder that such frustrated spirits find themselves in the hands of the doctor, the public health nurse, the judge and even the jailer? Such, at least, are some of the problems which the migration of a people with one cultural mentality to a community with a different mentality present to modern medical and legal science. Clearly a legal education which, in the traditional Anglo-American custom, restricts itself to the study of nothing but Anglo-American positive law, after the manner of Austin, Thayer and Judge Emeritus Learned Hand, cannot meet contemporary legal problems. Only a legal education which relates positive law to the underlying cultural mentalities of the people in our cities to whom it is applied can hope therefore to prepare lawyers, judges and statesmen to meet today's diseases of the body politic. The same, needless to say, is true also of the education of the teacher and doctor if they are to heal the wounds of the spirit and of the body of men.

There remains a third respect in which cultural mentalities are important for medical science. This respect becomes evident when one notes that certain diseases of modern Western man do not occur in so-called primitive man.

SOME DISEASES OF MODERN WESTERN SOCIETIES

During the aforementioned visit to Mexico City in 1949, the writer met one morning with Dr. Salvador Zubiran and Dr. Ignacio Chávez in the latter's office in the Instituto Nacional de Cardiologia. Our appointment was for 9 o'clock. The clock showed that it was two minutes of nine. Commenting upon this fact I said, "Of the many appointments during my three weeks in Mexico City, this is the only one in which all participants have been on time. I presume this is because my previous appointments have been, for the most part, with humanists, whereas this appointment is with scientists in a scientific laboratory." Dr. Chávez, who is one of the leading authorities in the world on diseases of the heart and arteries, replied: "You are probably right in saying that the modern scientific mentality is the reason for the discrepancy you describe. I am not sure, however, that this mentality is a good thing. I say this because autopsies, made here in this laboratory, of Indians who have spent their lives carrying heavy loads from the valley of Mexico City [which is 7,500 feet above sea level] up the sides of the surrounding mountains, show that their arteries often possess the elasticity of those of young people. European pathologists who make these autopsies simply cannot believe their eyes; there is so little if any hardening of the arteries." Dr. Chávez added that when Mexico's native Indians receive a little modern Western education and enter modern politics they also achieve the distinction of having extensive hardening of the arteries after the manner of good modern Westerners.

In 1953 the writer told Dr. James B. Hannah, who practices medicine in Northern Rhodesia, of Dr. Chávez's observations. Dr. Hannah replied that the same phenomena occurred with his African negroes.

In its issue of December 8, 1955, *The Listener* of London printed a broadcast by Dr. J. N. Morris (3) of the British Medical Research Council. This published report bore the title, "Coronary Thrombosis: A Modern Epidemic," and referred to the following facts. First, reliable vital statistics in Great Britain show that the death rate from this disease among men between fifty-five and sixty-four years of age was "about ten per cent higher than that of women" a century ago, whereas today it is about ninety per cent and "is worsening." Second, comparative studies in different cultural areas demonstrate that peoples in underdeveloped regions "suffer less, and apparently much less, coronary thrombosis than do more advanced, more prosperous, western peoples." For example, Morris adds, the rural Guatemalans, the Bantus of South Africa, the Okinawans and the rural Japanese "have little coronary thrombosis." Also Jews from Western Europe in contemporary Israel suffer a great deal, whereas those from the Middle East and North Africa "do not—or not yet." Similarly the United States, Canada, Australia and New Zealand have a higher incidence of this disease than does Great Britain which in turn has more than Denmark and Norway.

These observations make another conclusion evident. The modern mathematically exact scientific mentality and social behavior, expressing itself through modern medical science, cures certain diseases only at the cost of creating others. One escapes typhoid, malaria and dysentery to be sure, but acquires ulcers, hardening of the arteries and coronary thrombosis in their stead.

Why does the modern Western mentality have this debit side of its medical balance sheet? An examination of the mentality of the African, the Chinese and the humanistic Spanish Indian Mexican, who are fearful of absolute commitments and somewhat casual about appointments,[1] throws considerable light upon this question. The Spanish-Mexican word which expresses this mentality and its attendant social behavior is *"mañana."* The corresponding Cantonese word is *"wock-jeh." Mañana* means "Let's put it off until tomorrow or do it when we feel like doing it, if we possibly can." *"Wock-jeh"* means "Perhaps." The southern Italian word, we have noted, is *"pazienza."*

If one asks the reason for the *wock-jeh-mañana-pazienza* mentality, or for any other norm of the unwesternized native's behavior, the answer will be as follows: Such a way of thinking and behaving is good because it "brings man into harmony with nature," or "preserves the cosmic equilibrium." Two points are to be noted in this type of answer. First, the individual thinks of himself as immersed in nature and as responsible for the preservation of the harmony or the equilibrium of nature. Second, goodness and health are conceived as accepting and conforming to nature's rhythm and balance. In practice, this means restoring the harmony or equilibrium when nature gives an immediately felt warning that a disharmony or disequilibrium is occurring; evil and disease result when such warnings are not heeded. As Sigerist has noted, "When a

1 Referring again to Mexican-Americans, Dr. Saunders (7, pp. 105, 107) reports, "School teachers and employers often feel frustrated at their inability to get school children and employees to report at the appointed time."

Navaho . . . feels 'bad all over,' it is because he 'fell out of harmony with the forces of nature' " (8, p. 199). To any primitive person, nature's warnings that something is wrong are not ambiguous. They show concretely in one's feelings; one "feels bad all over." When such emotional irritation is felt, the non-Westernized native interprets this as nature telling him that it is time for a siesta and a little patience with respect to when the job gets done. Furthermore, empirical observation shows that the moments when emotive irritations come cannot be predicted. Consequently, if one is to heed nature's warnings, future commitments must be fastened to a *"wock-jeh,"* a "Perhaps," and made and met with the *"mañana"* attitude of mind. Such a philosophy of nature and of social relations is hardly conducive to an inner conflict or to a physiological strain upon the vascular system.

The need to observe natural phenomena if one is to keep oneself in harmony with nature is also necessary. The most obvious recurrent phenomenon of nature is the sequence of darkness and brightness which is night and day. Consequently, to harmonize with nature tends to mean getting up when the sun rises and going to bed when it sets. The Sicilians express this belief in a proverb: "Sleep is the ordinance of God, who has made night to follow day" (9, p. 43).

The first effect of Western commercial society upon non-Western peoples is to provide kerosene. It immediately disrupts the traditional physiological and social habits by providing oil lamps which lengthen the brightness of day for work and conversation far beyond the natural day's span. Here we probably have the first step down the road to hardening of the arteries which modern Western ways impose upon pre-modern man. The subsequent steps have their source, however, in a different factor. This factor becomes evident when we examine the mentality which brings everyone to a nine o'clock appointment at two minutes of nine.

The individuals concerned must have mechanically exact watches or there must be frequently spaced public clocks. Moreover, these watches and clocks must be socially and exactly synchronized. For this synchronization there must be an absolute standard which is set by a social convention. This social convention requires the use of the Western law of contract with its legislated statutes applying equally to all men. Also this absolute standard, set by the contractual legal mentality, must be located somewhere. It is not an accident that Greenwich is in the modern European western portion of the world or that the Bureau of Standards is in Washington.

Furthermore, the un-Westernized native with merely nature's emotive warnings and immediately sensed dawns and dusks is quite incapable of even grasping, to say nothing of determining, the legally sanctioned Greenwich standard of time. The so-called practical man with nothing but his ordinary common sense concepts and knowledge is equally incapable of this. Only an astronomer who is a mathematical physicist and who is equipped with a very refined telescope constructed upon the basis of the principles of mathematical mechanics and optics can determine the time of the Greenwich standard.

Mathematical physics requires a quite different way of thinking about time and space, or anything else, from that which exhibits itself in a time sequence that is based upon one's gross aesthetic sense of day and night or one's comfortable or uncomfortable emotive feelings concerning when it is time to get up or to take a siesta. Newton, at the beginning of his *Principia*, which laid the foundations of the modern Western mentality, noted this radical difference between immediately sensed and felt time and the time of mathematical physics in which modern man lives with his quantitatively exact social engagements. The latter time, which Newton quite appropriately termed "mathematical time," "flows uniformly" and is the same for all people on the surface of the earth. Immediately sensed, or physiologically felt time, Newton noted, does not flow uniformly and is one thing for one person and a different thing for another.[2]

Need one be surprised, therefore, that modern man, whose mentality and social engagements derive from Newton's quantitatively and publicly precise mathematical way of thinking about time, is able to make and keep exact appointments, whereas people, whose mentality and social behavior derive from directly sensed and emotively felt time, find this difficult if not impossible? Need one be surprised also that when the former type of cultural mentality and behavior causes its adherents to ignore nature's warnings by way of the emotively and bodily felt irritations, that diseases of the heart and arteries occur for such people which do not occur for so-called primitive people with their different conception of time and of social engagements? Should one wonder also, after driving the human emotional and physiological being through a cold-blooded time schedule in which the mechanical clock's hands stand over one's head like a policeman's club in total disregard of one's physiological and emotional feelings and warnings, that nature rebels with a physical explosion that

[2] For an account of the effect of these two ways of thinking about time upon the Spanish-Mexicans in the United States, see Saunders (7, pp. 104-111, 117-122).

blows one's heart or arteries apart, or with an epidemic of emotional explosions that fill the doctors' offices, the divorce courts and the ever-increasing number of hospitals to overflowing with chronic neurotics?

Consider by way of contrast the sense of time and its emotive effects of a non-Western mentality. Two examples will show how it operates. A few years ago Mr. Francis S. F. Liu was a colleague of the writer on the faculty of the Yale Law School. Mr. Liu was trained in both the classical Confucian Chinese way of thinking and dispute settling and in the Western way, having first been educated in classical Chinese and then in Western law in both the United States and Europe. Returning from Europe to China after President Chiang Kai-shek's introduction of the Western law of contract, Mr. Liu started to practice law in Shanghai in the Western manner. Two things happened—one of legal, the other of medical interest—both intimately connected. Legally, Mr. Liu's attempt to practice Western law resulted in the loss of his Chinese clients. Medically, it brought him home in the evening psychologically and physically exhausted. After locating the cause of his loss of clients in their persisting Confucian Chinese mentality, notwithstanding President Chiang Kai-shek's introduction of Western legal ways, Mr. Liu met his predicament by returning to the classical Confucian Chinese mode of dispute settling by means of delicate mediation between the disputants through a third party. This type of legal practice not only brought in the Chinese clients but also enabled Mr. Liu to go through the day's meetings with his clients in the exceedingly slow and apparently irrelevant manner of inquiring at great length about their families and leisurely drinking frequent cups of tea. The interesting psychological and medical result was that Mr.

Liu went home at night as emotionally and physically relaxed and refreshed as when he arrived at his office in the morning. Moreover, disputes for the most part were settled in the Confucian manner by the parties themselves without going to court or other recourse to litigation.

Consider also the negroes of Northern Rhodesia. Dr. Hannah told the writer that he had never met one who knew his age. If in the late afternoon Dr. Hannah asks the boy who takes care of the horses whether he had watered them, the reply is in one of three forms if he has done so: (a) "Yes," with the boy's arm pointing straight up to the sky above his head; (b) "Yes," with the arm pointing to the West, or (c) "Yes," with the arm pointing to the East. The first of these three arm pointings means, "I watered them approximately at mid-day"; the second means, "I watered them sometime in the afternoon"; and the third means that "I watered them sometime in the morning." Dr. Hannah added that so far as he was able to determine these were about the only temporal distinctions which his boy was able to comprehend. The same absence of fine distinctions applies to the Africans' conception of different days. In one African tribe, the word for "yesterday" and the word for "tomorrow" is the same word. Similarly in the ancient Vedic hymns of the Hindus, the word for dawn and that for dusk is identical (4).

One is reminded of a contemporary American negro, known to all followers of professional baseball as Satchel Paige. His Christian name was acquired because Mr. Paige refused to grow old, with the result that the teams for which he played died before he did and forced him to acquire a valise to carry his equipment over the decades from one club to another. In recent years he was a relief pitcher for the Cleveland Indians and the St. Louis

Browns. Some of the more serious anthropologists have investigated his ways and his mentality. They have found that the newspapermen, notwithstanding countless efforts, could never obtain from Old Satch a satisfactory statement of his age. Yet his answer was quite clear; he was "forty-nine," meaning, of course, "approximately"; and forty-nine it remained in the sports' writers' reports over the years. During the time when the white ball-players and the university educated Jackie Robinson's knees, muscles and reflexes gave out at the age of the middle thirties or at an occasional forty-one, forty-two or forty-three, Old Satch went on pitching year after year—a perennial forty-nine.

This miraculous constancy of his age did not bother him very much. Nor was he troubled during the games as he sat in the bull pen with the other pitchers awaiting the inevitable moment, which was frequent on the St. Louis Browns, when the enemy bats would start to connect with the starting pitcher's pitches and Old Satch would know that the time had come for him to make his cool, leisurely and casual shamble from the bull pen to the pitcher's mound. Like the Lord Krishna's advice to Arjuna on the battlefield, as recorded in the Hindu's beloved *Bhagavad-gita,* Old Satch entered into the battle, as did other men, but with "non-attachment." Nor did he wear out his nerves, his disposition or his arteries in physical uneasiness, shifting the seat of his trousers from one splinter to another on the bench when in the bull pen. Instead, his manager, undoubtedly sensing Satchel's divine Buddhist-like serenity, provided him with a rocking chair in which he rocked leisurely back and forth, complacently watching the others do the worrying and the work. When some inquisitive reporter, with the tact of a modern State Department official, tried to shake Old Satch out of his good-natured equanimity by asking this ace reliever what his age was or why he didn't show a little more hustle, Old Satch would reply, "Don't you worry yo' head, Suh. Old Satch is not goin' to git himself mixed up with that old rascal Time."

The moral seems clear. The pre-modern mentality has its advantages as well as its liabilities for medical science. Perhaps there will be no end to our overcrowded hospitals filled with the emotionally starved and disturbed, not to mention the schizophrenics and incurably insane, as there may be no cure of diseases of the vascular system until the modern mathematically and mechanically precise and socially exacting mind incorporates into and reconciles within itself the more intuitive, emotive and impressionistically aesthetic values and ways of feeling, thinking and behaving of so-called primitive man and of the sages of the classical East. Certainly the diseases peculiar to modern man suggest a very real sense in which so-called primitive man is the true modern and we are the outmoded and misbehaving barbarians.

In any event, both medicine and men ignore facts of their peril. Hence it cannot be said too often that a sense of inner peace, a feeling of irritation or the basic philosophical way of thinking about time is just as much a fact to which medicine must adjust itself, if it is to be scientific, as is a patient's blood pressure, the hydrogen ion concentration of that blood or the chemistry of the bacteria in a polluted water supply. In fact, the philosophical concept of time, accepted unconsciously by both doctor and patient, may be the major cause of the high blood pressure. But when the cause of a disease is philosophical, the cure also must be philosophical. Concretely, this may very well mean that in prescribing a specific drug to alleviate the pain from the calcified arteries of a given patient, the physician of tomorrow will also call in that patient's children and prescribe for them a new, scientifically verified philosophical way of thinking about time, which harmoni ously embraces its emotively felt and its mathematically constructed components. In short, to become aware of the bearing of cultural mentalities upon medical science is to realize that the doctor, if he is to remain scientific, must draw upon research of the cultural anthropologist and the philosopher of both modern science and non-modern cultures.

REFERENCES

1. Child, Irvin L.: *Italian or American? The Second Generation in Conflict.* New Haven: Yale University Press, 1943.
2. Maine, Sir Henry S.: *Ancient Law.* London: John Murray, 1908.
3. Morris, J. N.: Coronary Thrombosis: A Modern Epidemic. *The Listener, 54*:995-996, 1955.
4. Muller, F. Max, ed.: *The Sacred Books of the East,* Vol. 32, Vedic Hymns. Oxford: Clarendon Press, 1891, pp. 241-245.
5. Nasmith, David: *Outline of Roman History.* London: Butterworths, 1890.
6. Pound, Roscoe: Toward a New Jus Gentium. In Northrop, ed.: *Ideological Differences and World Order.* New Haven: Yale University Press, 1948, pp. 1-17.
7. Saunders, Lyle: *Cultural Differences and Medical Care.* New York: Russell Sage Foundation, 1954.
8. Sigerist, Henry E.: *A History of Medicine,* Vol. I, Primitive and Archaic Medicine. New York: Oxford University Press, 1951.
9. Williams, Phyllis H.: *South Italian Folkways in Europe and America.* New Haven: Yale University Press, 1938.

MENTAL ILLNESS AND ACCULTURATION[1]

By Alexander H. Leighton, M.D.

INTRODUCTION

THE CENTRAL theme to be developed in these pages asserts that acculturation, when rapid and extensive, has a damaging effect on mental health. For example, natives of the Belgian Congo are now changing from their own way of life to patterns of European industry (6, 7, 8). If this occurs swiftly, then according to our thesis there will be a rise in mental illness among them.

There is a similarity in this to what has happened in some instances with regard to organic illness. As is well known, many groups such as Eskimos and American Indians have been decimated by the importation of tuberculosis and other "civilized" diseases to which they had little immunity. With mental illness, it is of course not a question of transmitting a disease as such. No germ is passed over. The process is, rather, an upset in equilibrium and may be likened to the effects of shifting from sea level to

1 Grateful acknowledgment is made to Charles C. Hughes for invaluable help in the preparation of this paper. Thanks are also to be expressed to the American Philosophical Society for a grant to return after a fifteen-year period to the Eskimo community used as an illustration in this chapter.

high altitude. People can live in good health at incredible elevations on the windy Andes, but if they move up too quickly from the coast to heights they are apt to become exceedingly ill due to disturbances in their physiological equilibrium. On the other hand, if the change is made slowly, bodily adjustments take place without the appearance of distressing symptoms. It is suggested that rapid acculturation has a similar effect on psychological equilibrium.

In making these observations on the destructive effect of the European and American way of life on other peoples, it is well to note that not all contacts result in organic disease and, similarly, no claim is made that all contacts are damaging to mental health. In some instances just the opposite is the case. However, it is thought that acculturation can, and frequently does, produce a decline in mental health and the emphasis here will be on indicating some reasons.

There has always been acculturation since the beginning of civilization. The different life-ways of different societies have been affecting each other as long as there has been such a thing as intergroup contact. But never before this century has the process been so rapid nor has it involved so many human beings in so many aspects of their lives. Hence the relationship of acculturation to mental health is assumed to be of correspondingly increased importance.

The topic is within the general framework of public health and preventive medicine and its study constitutes a meeting place of one branch of medicine (psychiatry) and one of the social sciences (anthropology). Its value lies in the hope it offers of devising methods for reducing and preventing mental illness. There is, however, no intention of deploring acculturation as such, nor asking for its repeal, even if this were possible. The point is rather one of management, so that the benefits acculturation confers on mankind may be achieved at a lower price in human suffering. The position entertained is analogous to that found in programs of better housing in crowded urban areas which do not imply any check on industrialization, however atrocious the slums.

There is one warning that must be sounded. Although some facts will be given, the discussions of cause and effect will be largely speculative. The crux of the presentation is an explanatory scheme which forms, it is hoped, some basis for steps toward better understanding of mental illness and its prevention. If the scheme is effective, it will, like other scientific theories, lead to research which will demolish and replace it with a better scheme.

MENTAL ILLNESS

"Mental Illness" are two words of broad meaning and vague limits. Because of the breadth, it is possible for people to use them and yet mean very different things. Just as the word "American" may refer to a New York policeman, a Louisiana 'Cajun housewife, or a nine year old Navaho shepherd boy, so "mental illness" can refer to a forgetful and disoriented old man, a young woman with two children who thinks she is the Virgin Mary, or a middle-aged stockbroker with ulcers. One hears the term used now to mean only psychoneurotic types of illness, and now to mean the total conglomeration of disturbed human behavior treated in state hospitals, including certain organic conditions such as paresis and epilepsy.

Aside from breadth, another difficulty is the fact that the boundary between mental health and mental illness is obscure. It is well to recognize that this is a problem which applies to all aspects of medicine, not just psychiatry. If one were to define health as the complete absence of every form of disease or disability, then it is doubtful that a single healthy human could be found anywhere. It is apparent, if one may venture to phrase it as a bull, that a certain amount of illness is normal. However, the question remains as to how much is normal; and different people for various purposes draw the dividing line at different points between absolute health and absolute illness. Even the specialists in psychiatry differ in this regard, as is often painfully demonstrated in conflicting court testimony.

When it comes to the outlook of specialist and non-specialist, the gap is even greater. Several research workers, particularly Shirley Star of the National Opinion Research Center (9), have made studies which indicate that the public in general may recognize only the grossest disturbances as mental illness and pass by, as normal, many types of behavior which virtually all psychiatrists would consider strongly indicative of disorder. Furthermore, such perceptions are apt to shift with circumstances. When international conditions are peaceful, the man who has spies on the brain is likely to be diagnosed as a paranoid schizophrenic much sooner than when there are wars and rumors of wars, although in both instances he may be equally ill.

These difficulties suggest the advisability of attempting to define at least roughly the area we propose to carpet in this chapter with "mental illness."

The terms will be used in a very broad sense and may be conceived as embracing seven major divisions.[2]

1. *Organic brain syndromes*—The commonest example

[2] These categories are based on the *Diagnostic and Statistical Manual, Mental Disorders,* prepared by the Committee on Nomenclature and Statistics of the American Psychiatric Association, Washington, 1952.

in this division is probably the behavior disturbances of old age, but there are also others such as delirium and the delayed effects of encephalitis.

2. *Mental deficiency*—This, of course, shows as low I.Q. when mental tests are applied. Included are many degrees from mild to severe.

3. *Psychoses*—These are the mental illnesses with extensive disorganization of personality and they typically require commitment to hospitals. Schizophrenia and manic-depressive states are examples.

4. *Psychophysiologic disturbances*—Here are placed organic disorders that have mainly an emotional basis. Some cases of peptic ulcer, skin disease and high blood pressure belong in this category. In a sense, this group is the opposite of organic brain syndromes. With the former, there is mainly organic cause with psychological result. Here the result is organic and the cause, at least in part, is psychological.

5. *Psychoneuroses*—These are conditions which impair people, yet do not, as a rule, take them out of the running in everyday life. Anxiety is a prominent characteristic, but the symptoms are protean, ranging from compulsive hand-washing to hypochondriasis.

6. *Personality trait disorders*—Conditions of this sort are often difficult to distinguish from the neuroses. They include such tendencies as general emotional instability or a persistent disposition to fly off the handle.

7. *Sociopathic disturbance*—This division undoubtedly overlaps a good deal with the other categories outlined but it is convenient in that it marks off all those whose behavior has, as its main characteristic, damage to society in some form. Many types of chronic trouble-makers, delinquents, alcoholics and drug addicts, may be grouped here

as people whose behavior is due to an underlying psychological disorder.

This, then, in very general terms, is the range of conditions included under mental illness. A pertinent question now is, how common are they? If we are going to consider the effects of acculturation on these various disorders, it is desirable to have some anchor point of orientation with regard to how frequently they occur.

There is no definitive answer to this question. National statistics show that each year 210,000 or more persons are admitted for the first time to mental hospitals. This may be compared to 14,665,195 who are admitted to hospitals of all sorts. An additional 70-80,000 are readmitted yearly to mental hospitals. Estimates based on records of service agencies suggest that there are about 9,000,000 persons in the United States suffering from mental disorders, 1.5 million of these being hospitalizable. This does not include 1.5 million mentally retarded individuals, of whom less than 10 per cent are in institutions (1, 2, 3).

The number of people known to agencies and getting treatment does not, of course, represent the total who are mentally ill. Hospital beds and other services available, community tolerance of mental illness and many more related factors tend to vary a good deal from one part of the country to another and to exert an influence on the number of known cases.

Let us therefore examine briefly the results of a survey designed to estimate true prevalence of symptoms of mental illness in a small town (5). It is assumed that this town is not unusual, but rather characteristic of many such that exist in Northeastern America.

TABLE I

Prevalence of Symptom Patterns. Per cent of Total Sample*
Showing Various Patterns

SYMPTOM PATTERN	PERCENTAGE
Brain Syndrome	3
Mental Deficiency	11
Psychosis	1
Psychophysiologic	77
Psychoneurotic	57
Personality Trait Disorder	12
Sociopathic Disturbance	17

* Since many individuals showed more than one symptom pattern, there is much overlap and the total far exceeds 100%. This table should be read:
"Brain syndrome 3% No brain syndrome 97%, etc."
The total number of individuals surveyed was 283.

The population is about 3,000 and a probability sample of a little less than 20 per cent of the adults was surveyed. The results are shown in Table I.

It should be noted that the table refers to patterns of symptoms not diagnoses. Furthermore, it does not distinguish between those whose lives are heavily impaired and those who are only very lightly affected. A general impression of degree of impairment may be indicated, however, by stating that when all these symptom groups are lumped together, 48 per cent of the adult population is estimated to be impaired to the extent that medical help would be advisable. Virtually all, however, are able to carry on their lives in some fashion, despite their symptoms and their disability. The survey did not include people currently in hospitals for mental illness.

Until other areas have been studied in a similar manner we cannot be sure, of course, that this sample is typical of North America, or even small towns in North America.

To sum up and conclude this section, a sketch has been given of the types of behavior disorder covered by the term "mental illness" and figures have been presented to suggest their frequency in our society. Although the figures may appear depressing, they are not necessarily static. They constitute a challenge to improve mental health and point up the need for public health effort, with particular reference to prevention.

ACCULTURATION

The boundaries of the term acculturation are about as vague and disputed as are those of mental health and mental illness.[3] There is, however, a central core of meaning that may be outlined.

The first time I recall hearing the word was on meeting that great and volcanic figure in anthropology, Bronislaw Malinowski. This was in the 1930's when he came to speak to the staff of the Psychiatric Clinic at Johns Hopkins and I was delegated to meet him at the station. He came along the platform and on spotting me as his reception committee he brandished a black, tightly wrapped Chamberlain type of umbrella, saying, "I hope you will pardon this symbol of British acculturation."

At the time, all I caught was that something had been said about culture and I thought he was apologizing with

[3] The Social Science Research Council Summer Seminar on Acculturation, 1953: "Acculturation: An Exploratory Formulation." *Am. Anthropol.*, *56* (No. 6), 1954.

a joke for an English cultural trait which—like spats—looked a little silly in the American context, much as horn-rimmed glasses, a straw hat and cigar might have seemed in England. It was later that I came to recognize that he was referring to the fact that he, a Pole, having moved to England, had changed in many ways from being a Pole to being an Englishman. He talked at some length about this afterward and spoke also of his friend, Joseph Conrad, another Pole with similar experience.

Acculturation, as it will be employed here, refers to the process in which the customs, knowledge, attitudes, values and material objects of one culture or way of life, become adopted in whole or in part by the people of another. Gaul was acculturated by the Romans, Britain by the Normans, Ireland by the English, the North American Indians by European settlers, to name a few instances. While not necessarily a one-way process—the settlers got lacrosse, maize and much else from the Indians—an outstanding feature of the world today is the fact that for vast numbers of people acculturation is mainly in one direction. The culture of Western Europe and North America—the North Atlantic civilization—is changing the life-ways of all sorts of different groups of people in all sorts of places. Such peoples are shifting from their traditional customs and outlook to patterns of behavior and feeling that embody our techniques in industry and agriculture, our material objects such as plumbing and airplanes, and our values—scientific, political, religious, ethical, legal and philosophic.

This is not to say that the recipient people are dropping everything old, or that they lack original contributions of their own. The contrary is the case. Moreover, the results of acculturation are often a pattern that is new, being different both from the native old way and from the North

Atlantic model. The main impetus, nevertheless, does come from the North Atlantic civilization and the people affected are undergoing an acculturation which is both extensive and essentially one-way.

In order to give a little more concreteness to this concept of acculturation, let us consider briefly one specific group, an Eskimo village on St. Lawrence Island, Alaska. The surrounding landscape of mountains, tundra, lakes and seacoast is for the most part empty of human beings. The village itself—composed of about 300 people—lies at the end of a gravel spit that sticks out into the Bering Sea, not far from Siberia.

Figure 1[4] shows one of the older men dressed in a rainproof parka made from walrus intestines and sewn with reindeer sinew. Underneath, in all probability, he is wearing furs. In contrast to this we see in Figure 2 the younger generation completely equipped in mail-order clothes. The difference, however, involves many things besides materials. The clothes of the older man are obtained through native skills—the skill of the hunter and the skill of the seamstress. The clothes of the children can only be obtained through cash and this means that the parents must have marketable products or wage-earning positions. Out of such a need come new pressures into village life, a heightened dependency on the outside world, and, in view of its limited economic possibilities, an urge to emigrate.

The difference in clothing implies more than economic factors; it also involves attitudes between the generations. These children do not look up to the older people in the same way their predecessors did twenty to thirty years ago.

[4] The photographs were taken by Dorothea C. Leighton and Charles C. Hughes in a village which they and the author have been studying for a number of years.

There is an alteration in feelings of respect and perceptions of wisdom, and with this an effect on the cohesion, communication, authority systems and sense of belonging in the village.

In Figures 3 and 4 old and new types of houses may be compared. Despite appearance, the old house is warm and can be heated with seal oil lamps. It is also made of materials that are for the most part locally available. The new house represents a considerable cash investment since the milled lumber has to come by steamer from great distances. This one was constructed the year its owner made $7,000 in trapping arctic foxes. Once built, it continues to demand cash, because it must be heated with kerosene or other imported oil, and it must be painted and kept in repair against severe weather conditions.

The new house also brings a different style of living. The floor use of the traditional house is shown in Figure 5. With the new house there are tables and chairs, and with these there are new motor habits, new manners, new attitudes between husband, wife and their children. There are also new kinds of recreation as can be seen from the radio and phonograph records in Figure 6. Such sources of vicarious entertainment present a contrast to the creation of music and poetry in the native style of singing with drums which is now passing away.

The point it is desired to emphasize is neither the advantages nor the disadvantages of these changes, but rather the widespread ramifications. Here we see in selected pictures physical manifestation of acculturation, but observation in the village shows that these have correspondences which interpenetrate virtually all aspects of the society.

This type of illustration from the Eskimo could be duplicated in hundreds of different cultural groups from

Alaska to Tierra del Fuego, in the Pacific Islands, and on the land mass of Asia. With such spread and variation, the question arises as to whether or not there are any universal features in the acculturation process.

There is here again no definitive answer but there are some indications. A few years ago a number of anthropologists at Cornell explored the question by comparing seven villages in widely different parts of the world.[5] The villages were located on the Navaho reservation in New Mexico, in Peru, Thailand, Burma, India, Japan, and Northeastern America. The latter, a sample of our own culture, was included as a point of reference. The anthropologists concluded that there were a limited number of rather striking patterns of change common to all these exceedingly different groups. Of these, the most salient for the purposes of this chapter is one that has to do with rate of change.

Rate of change varied considerably from one village to another and there appeared to be a relationship between rapid and extensive change on the one hand, and serious disorganization of the society on the other. By "disorganization" is meant the disruption of customs, communication, authority systems, cooperation and shared values, such that problems of morale are raised and there is actual threat to the group's existence. If change occurs slowly, that is, only a few items at a time, it seems that a society can generally adjust without widespread disruption of its functions. Families hold together, law and order are maintained, a recognizable moral code prevails, group decisions and cooperation are possible, and the economic base continues to be sufficient. When on the other hand change is too fast and extensive, there is multiplication of disruptive

[5] For a report on this see Leighton and Smith (4).

effects which set up self-perpetuating spirals of disorganization. Breaks in communication, for instance, interfere with the authority system which itself is already rocking from changes in values. Both these effects are in turn magnified by economic disturbances—and so on. The adaptive resources are thus taxed beyond their capacity and the society begins to fall apart. Our Navaho group was an example of this extreme.

The situation may be likened to rebuilding a house while living in it with your family. If the changes are made with some order and timing, it is possible, even if not comfortable, to live in the house and to have the use of its shelter, cooking, sleeping and plumbing facilities. If, on the other hand, the wreckers and the builders descend on the house all at once, maintenance of function and the process of change have a headlong collision that is likely to result in the family coming apart if it does not move out. In such a case, the home ceases to exist.

Like most analogies, this one can be misleading if carried too far. People are able not only to move out of a house, but also to move back again after it has been rebuilt. In the case of a society that is overwhelmed by change, there is no parallel opportunity.

To sum up and conclude, acculturation has been defined in descriptive terms and some illustrations given. It has also been pointed out that when acculturation occurs both extensively and rapidly, there is danger to the society.

At the same time one should underscore again the benefits of cultural change and the worth of the gifts which North Atlantic civilization is making to the rest of the world. Given undernourishment, high incidence of disease, early death, and threats to individual freedom, to name only a few items, acculturation has much to offer many

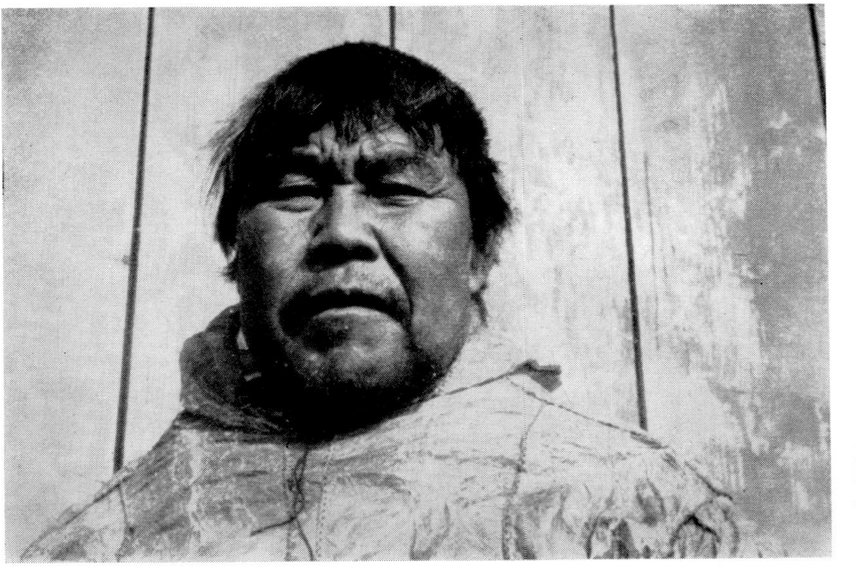

Fig. 1

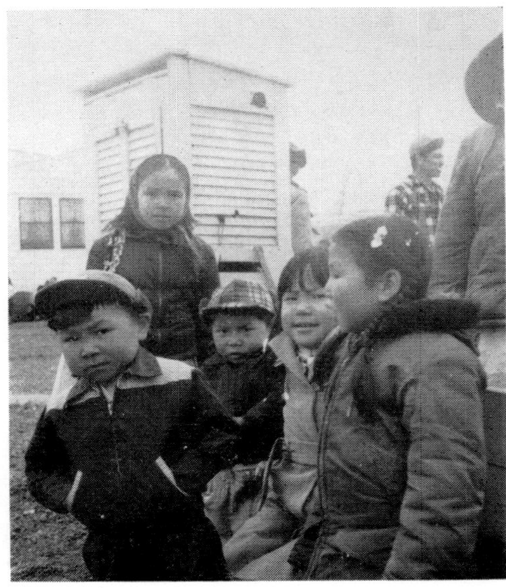

Fig. 2

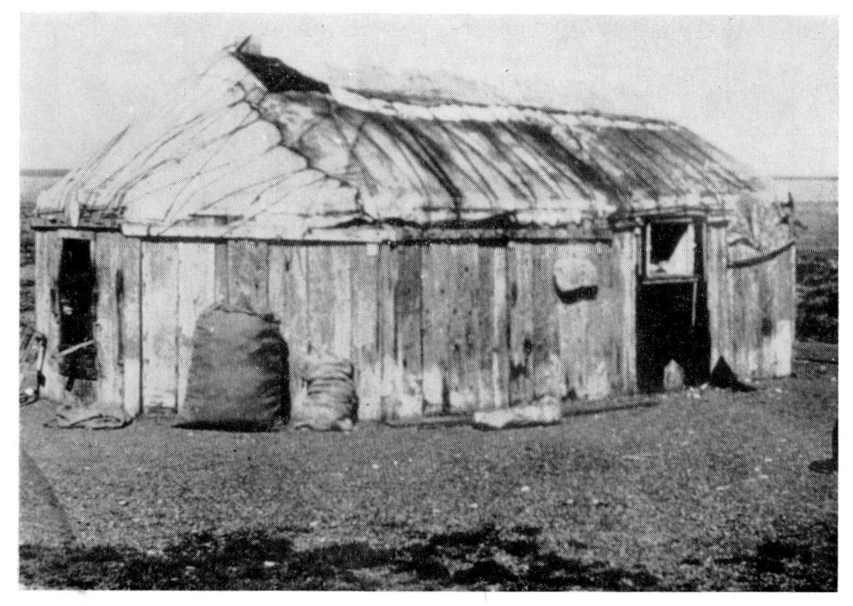

Fig. 3

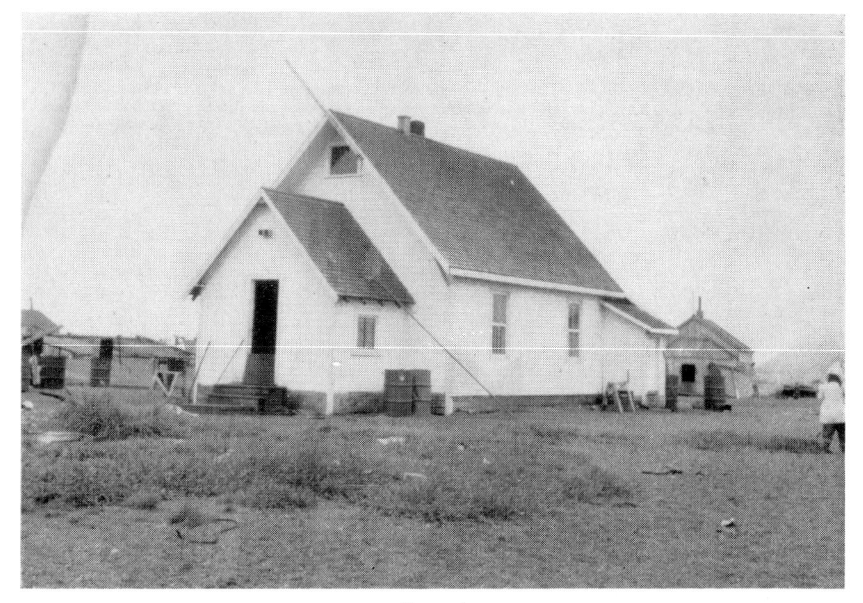

Fig. 4

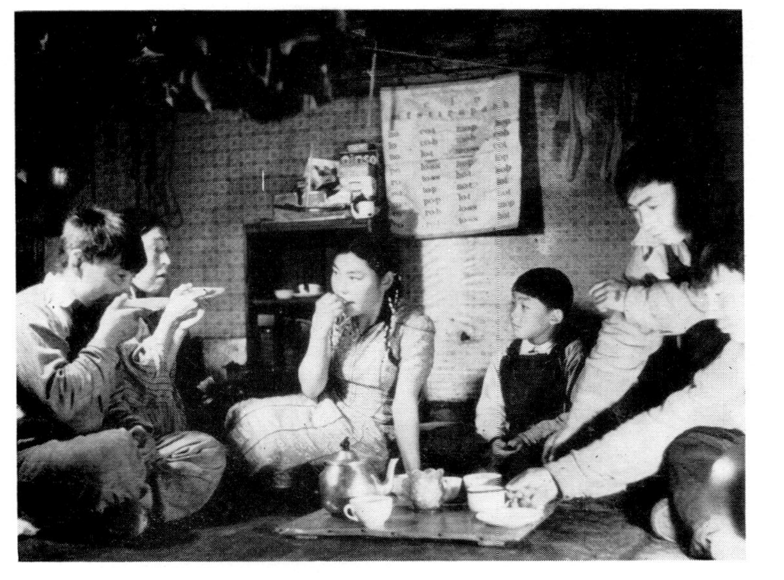

Fig. 5

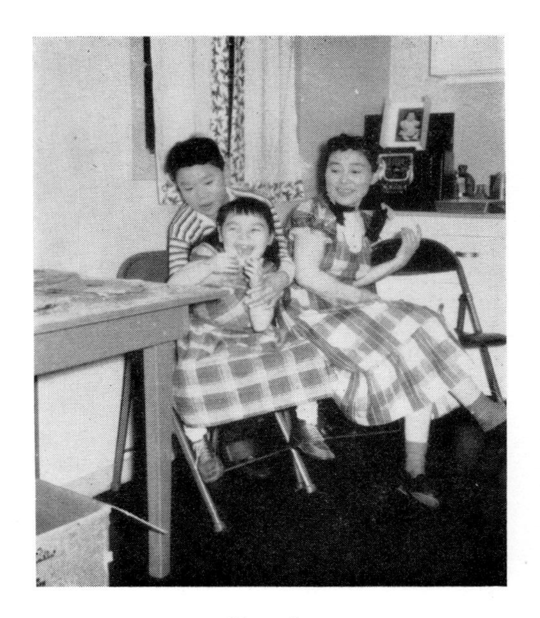

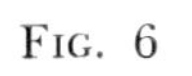

Fig. 6

peoples. The point is, however, that the relationship between change and social disorganization is such as to suggest that innovation is somewhat like a surgical operation. Both innovation and surgery are often desirable, even necessary, but they are nonetheless fraught with risk. In communities the danger is that too rapid acculturation may constitute a change that is too fast for the group to absorb, and as a result there may be failures in those functions upon which the welfare and survival of the group depend.

EFFECTS OF ACCULTURATION ON MENTAL HEALTH

The social disorganization which has been said to result when acculturation is too rapid and too extensive should not be confused with mental illness. Social disorganization refers to group functions, such as have been mentioned (maintaining law and order, providing opportunities for earning a living, or the rearing and education of children). These organizational aspects of society can break down under external pressure without the people concerned being mentally ill. However, the idea being put forward is that sustained social disorganization does lead to mental illness.

In approaching this thesis it is necessary to take a look at the general problem of cause in mental illness and the first point to stress in this connection is that causes are multiple. Any single case of mental illness is a complex process in which there are a number of major contributing factors, any one or all of which may be considered causal. A neurosis, for instance, may be based on predisposing factors that are hereditary, on malformation of personality due to infantile experience, and on precipitating strain in adult life. The same can be said for psychophysiological disorders such as ulcer and asthma, but here we must also add that there may be an organic element. A blow on the head that is followed by odd behavior might be considered a clear case of a single cause, yet even this is not a safe assumption. The patient's heredity, previous life experience, personality structure, and his perceptions regarding who gave the blow and why may all enter into determining whether or not he will show symptoms, and if so, what kind of symptoms.

In view of this welter of considerations, it is convenient to think of causes in terms of three major—even if overlapping—categories.

1. *Constitutional*—These are built into the organism and are primarily hereditary.

2. *Physical damage*—Here may be included injury to the brain as from a blow, or from a poison such as lead, or from infections, or from a deprivation in diet. An example of the latter is pellagra, a combination of skin disease, diarrhea, and dementia due to lack of certain vitamins.

3. *Psychological experience*—This may be considered in two parts: (a) Emotional strains during growth and development which result in deformity of personality; (b) Emotional strains on the grown personality which result in its disintegration. The former may be illustrated by mishaps in infancy and childhood such as not having a mothering person. The latter can be seen in such traumatic experiences as battle, loss of love, or conditions which tend to shatter one's self-respect.

Referring now to social disorganization, it would be hard to show that this has any constant relationship to greater frequency of mental illness through increased breeding of people with defective heredity. One can imagine special cases in which the breakdown of the sociocultural system leads to the disappearance of marriage taboos, birth control methods, or segregation practices, so that there is more reproduction by grossly defective individuals. This, however, can hardly be considered a prominent and widespread characteristic of social disorganization.

Physical damage, by contrast, is apt to be increased in almost any disorganized society. A group that is failing in its functions offers more chance of accident, physical strain, infections, toxic substances, and inadequate nutrition for the embryo, the child, the adult, and the aged.

In noting this, it is realized that many underdeveloped areas in the world have these conditions as endemic, and one of the promises of acculturation is to overcome them and raise the standard of living. This, however, does not prevent the process of change, if it leads to disorganization, from making these adverse conditions even worse, regardless of the purpose and nature of the change.

The main effect of disorganization comes to bear at the level of psychological cause. Referring to the arc of life from birth to death we may note the impact of disorganization at three main points: in the formative years, during maturity, and in later years.

In the formative years the personality is being laid down and is susceptible to acquiring basic patterns which will last through the rest of the individual's existence. At such a time disruption of family life, confused values, excessively inconsistent behavior on the part of parents and brothers and sisters, disjunctions between what one is trained to expect and the realities of life as one finds them, discrepancies between the orientation of the family and the world outside the family—all these can generate basic anxieties, perduring apprehensions, and maladaptive and misfiring psychological defenses. Thus both in earliest infancy and at a later stage of building patterns of expectation with regard to interpersonal relations outside the family, a disorganized and confused society can leave a permanent mark disposing toward mental illness on the personalities growing up in such a situation.

During maturity, the stresses of poorly functioning society can add to the strains of living so that, whether or not predisposition has been laid down in the development of personality, strains are overwhelming and lead to symptom formation on their own.

In later years, with the decline of resources the effect of stress from a disorganized society can be even more severe on the individual. It has often been demonstrated that old people develop mental symptoms in a confused and otherwise stressful environment, yet lose them again when circumstances improve. It seems that although they are capable of normal function, they have reduced reserves of tolerance for difficulties.

We may suppose, therefore, that rapid acculturation leads to social disorganization which in turn affects both *disposition* toward, and *precipitation of* mental disorders. The disease categories affected range from some types of organic brain disorders, through psychoses, psychoneuroses, personality trait disorders to sociopathic behavior—in short, all of the categories outlined in the beginning of this chapter as making up mental illness, with the possible exception of mental deficiency.

The potentially adverse effects of acculturation do not, however, stop here. The opportunities for treatment also must be considered. In a society with adequate organization and a stable culture there are usually resources for coping with some of the symptoms of mental illness and for reducing them. Through wise-men, religious leaders, professional healers, and others, there are often what amounts to counselling, opportunities for ventilation, and numerous customs and institutions which help an individual to deal with his inacceptable tendencies and to direct, displace or neutralize his symptoms. There are, in short, brakes on symptom formation and symptom perpetuation. These are not, obviously, wholly successful, but it may be supposed that they have some effect. In a disorganized society such brakes are very weak, if they exist at all.

CONCLUSION

By way of general summary it may be said that all societies have endemic mental illness due to factors that are in part constitutional, in part due to noxious physical agents, and in part arising from psychological experience. No culture provides complete protection. If acculturation occurs rapidly and extensively in a society, that society is apt to pass, at least for a time, into a state of disorganization in which it begins to fail in many of its vital functions. If the disorganization lasts any length of time, there is consequent increase in the occurrence of noxious physical agents and of adverse psychological experience for individual members, with the general result that there is a rise in mental disorders.

All of this adds up to the suggestion that rate of acculturation is a problem of some interest in public health. If the idea of preventive medicine is applicable to psychiatry, then here is a region for study with a view to some psychological engineering to neutralize as many as possible of the undesirable effects of too rapid change. The situation has implications not only for physicians, but also for the planners of change, whether these be in the governments of countries that are deliberately trying to adopt major aspects of North Atlantic culture, or whether they be in our own programs of aid for underdeveloped areas. These implications include the desirability of giving thought to the rate of change already in process in any given society and to the effect of an additional load. It puts emphasis on understanding what is in progress *before* an innovation is introduced, and it gives particular importance to questions of *timing*. Otherwise, no matter how worthy the goal, there may be serious effects, including damage to mental health.

In the course of these pages the word "change" has been used many times. This reflects the fact that acculturation is one aspect of a still larger process. It is a particular type of change in human life-ways. Another major type of change is one that goes on, self-generated, in the North Atlantic culture itself. Although different in origin from acculturation, it has many of the same characteristics, including the capacity to produce disorganization. We are, therefore, exposed to similar influences with regard to mental illness and have among ourselves the same problems of prevention as are found in rapidly acculturating peoples. There is reason, therefore, to think about the possibilities of controlling such change—*of pacing it so as to humanize it.* Public health and preventive psychiatry have a concern in this, much as a sanitary engineer might have an interest in city alterations that disturb old drainage and yet do not lay new pipes fast enough.

In concluding, I would like to suggest that these considerations extend beyond the limits of the mental health field—of clinically defined illness. Among the ingredients of mental illness are anxiety, hostility, hatred, and irrational addiction to suspicions, fixed ideas, even delusions. The objects of these dangerous attitudes are of course people, often groups of people. Hence in the upheavals of acculturation and allied trends in change we have the seeds of maladaptive reactions that are destructive to human living and to peace. One can imagine a changing society as being something like a spinning fly-wheel, which, if the speed becomes too great, starts to fly apart, and may smash the engine house along with itself.

But if this does not happen, there are marvelously constructive possibilities for an ever-expanding and better way of life. Rostand's Cyrano de Bergerac was told that, if like Don Quixote he tilted at windmills, he would get dashed down into the mud by the swinging sails. He answered with the other possibility. He said, "or up among the stars," and I think this is also our choice.

REFERENCES

1. Clausen, John A. and Yarrow, Marian Radke: The Impact of Mental Illness on the Family. *J. Soc. Issues, 11* (No. 4), 1955.
2. *Group for the Advancement of Psychiatry Published Reports,* No. 7. Vol. 1, 1947-1951.
3. Gruenberg, Ernest and Bellin, Seymour S.: The Impact of Mental Disease on Society. In: Leighton, Alexander H., Clausen, John A., and Wilson, Robert N. (eds.), *Explorations in Social Psychiatry*. New York: Basic Books, 1957.
4. Leighton, Alexander H. and Smith, Robert J.: A Comparative Study of Social and Cultural Change. *Proc. Am. Philo. Soc., 99* (No. 2), 1955.
5. Leighton, Dorothea C.: The Distribution of Psychiatric Symptoms in a Small Town. *Am. J. Psychiat., 112* (No. 9), 1956.
6. Maquet, J. J.: Modern Evolution of African Population in the Belgian Congo. *Africa, 19*:265, 1949.
7. Peigneux, F.: Le Logement du Travailleur Urbain au

Congo Belge et au Ruanda-Urundi. *Problèmes d'Afrique Centrale, 6*:175-189, 1953.
8. Pendleton, Robert L.: The Belgian Congo: Impressions of a Changing Region. *Geog. Rev., 39*:371-400, 1949.
9. Star, Shirley: *Popular Thinking in the Field of Mental Health.* From a mimeographed report of the National Opinion Research Center, University of Chicago.

ACCULTURATION IN RELATION TO CONCEPTS OF HEALTH AND DISEASE

By Raymond Firth, Ph.D.[1]

THIS lecture is a challenge. Anthropology is a well-established scientific discipline, or set of disciplines, of growing reputation, dealing with various aspects of human society and human culture from a comparative point of view. Very recently anthropologists have been brought into relation with medical work, especially in what have been called the under-developed areas. But I am reminded here of a remark of Jean Cocteau about poetry, when he was installed not long ago as a member of the French Academy. He said characteristically, "I know that poetry is essential. But I do not know what it is essential for!" Now much the same is still true of ideas about anthropology in relation to medicine. Many of us are convinced that anthropology is of vital importance to medical studies, especially in fields of rapid acculturation. But it is not so easy to explain just how necessary, until we have done much more work upon the subject. We anthropolo-

[1] I am grateful to Dr. Anne Burgess, Mrs. Margot Jefferys and Mr. Maurice Freedman for helpful comment on various points in this lecture, and to Dr. Paul Fejos for his great interest and encouragement.

gists sometimes may have to be cautious lest some of our more enthusiastic medical friends flatter us into thinking we are greater than we know, and appeal to us for solutions of their more refractory problems.

For this they have excuse, for some of their problems are indeed refractory. As doctors they are faced by a paradox. In many parts of the world Western science and Western medicine are being rapidly introduced, along with many other benefits of modern technology and administration. Great sums, provided by foundations, international organizations, and governments—especially by the United States, with its usual generosity in such matters—are poured out annually for preventive and curative medicine. Hospitals are being built, health and maternity services established, skilled assistance given. And yet in these vast populations of high birth rate, high mortality rate, suffering from disease and misery which are capable of great alleviation by modern medical science, there is a block.

The people seek health and want to avoid disease. They want to be cured of their ills. Yet they are often unwilling to go to the hospital; they are careless about treatment; they refuse to take elementary precautions which the doctor recommends; they will not change their food habits; they prefer their own midwives and medicine men. They show no resistance to many other Western items. They accept the movies and the radio eagerly; they take to candies, to alcohol and even to tobacco, without a thought for their digestions or their lung cancer; the men buy sportswear and jazzy ties for themselves, and seductive perfume and lipstick for their girl-friends. They accept these forms of acculturation without any effort at persuasion. Their acculturation is not spread evenly over the whole range of their behavior. It is often most defective in regions of health, where one might think it would be most receptive. Clearly there is something in their notions of health which needs looking into. But clearly also these notions are related to other kinds of ideas they have—about the good things of life, about human relationships that matter, about ways of spending time and money.

This is where the challenge—or the question—to the anthropologist begins. I have some sympathy with those medical men who are antipathetic to anthropology and the allied social sciences, who ask only to be allowed to get on with their own job, the prevention and cure of disease and the maintenance of healthy populations. But what do they propose to do about this paradox, that people who seem to want to get well or keep well do not seem to be at all anxious to take the benefits which the Western-trained medical man wishes to offer them? We may say that the people must just learn in time to accept the new ways. But do they learn? And how does one make people learn? These are not easy questions to answer. They face us in our own society. There are very important practical problems here which cannot be dodged—how to make the best use of the medical resources expended, in men, money and equipment; how to develop a medical organization in such a way as to let it go *with* the stream of acculturation, of changing ideas and behavior patterns of the people, not against the stream; how to match modern scientific standards of health practice with local attitudes so that they meet at some point and do not grow further and further apart.

There are also basic theoretical problems in exploring the nature of human personality. The idea of health is an aspect of personality or, in other words, a way of conceiving of its positive functioning. This functioning goes on at different levels. It occurs, largely unconsciously, at the bodily level; it occurs, with a much greater degree of consciousness, at the mental level. And the two are linked together and influence one another very intricately. But a personality, even an animal personality, does not function in isolation. It operates in a social context, in relation to other personalities with shared interests.

There is, then, a social level of health, this also being subtly related to the others. It is this notion, I think, that is embodied in the World Health Organization's definition of health as a state of complete physical, mental and social well-being, and not merely the absence of disease and infirmity. This definition has certain difficulties which I will mention later. But it expresses an important truth—that one cannot understand the body without reference also to the mind, and that body and mind have full meaning only in relation to society. Of course to put the notions of health and personality in terms of different levels, or systems, is a convention. This is just one way of describing in a useful conceptual frame what are most complex and subtle phenomena. But using this particular frame, we are concerned to know how acculturation, the acquisition of new cultural forms, tends to produce changes in a people's ideas of bodily, mental and social well-being, and how such changes in ideas in turn react upon the way in which other new cultural elements are accepted. This is stating the problem very crudely, because acculturation is a very complex notion.

But what I am concerned with primarily here is to show how ideas about the well-being of the human personality, and mainly the physical well-being, respond to, or resist acculturative forces—changes in the medical and non-medical fields. I want to make clear too, how, when we consider these issues, the approach of anthropology, particularly social anthropology, is important and at times essential.

But first let me take a simple example, from my personal experience, of the way in which body, mind and society are related in illness.

In a remote South Pacific island, inhabited by less than 2,000 still fairly primitive Polynesians, a young woman is ill. She has a severe pain in the lower ribs. A local expert in curing illness is called in, and I go with him at his invitation. The house is full of relatives and neighbors, the patient sitting among them with bowed head, in evident distress, and supported by them. The practitioner asks about the symptoms, then calls for coconut oil. He pours a little out into the palm of his hand, and then gently rubs it on the patient's back and side. As he does so, he calls loudly on guardian spirits to turn to the patient, to help in her recovery, and to drive away impeding influences. Then he puts his lips to the girl's side, and sucks vigorously, afterwards spitting, to expel any noxious elements. Then he begins to massage the patient down her back, bunching his fingers together with much manipulation, as if to break down adhesions, and asking just where the pain is located. He intersperses these movements by blowing gently on the spot identified. Both the hand and the breath of the practitioner are believed to have power and healing effect. Then food is given to the patient, and she is urged to eat. But the pain has not abated. The practitioner says "The illness is not over."

He is a professional spirit-medium also, and he now announces that a spirit is about to enter him. His body writhes; one shoulder and then the other moves forward, with muscles rippling under the skin. After about ten seconds he has passed into a state of possession, or dissociation of a moderate kind. He turns to me with bright wide-open eyes and the vacant smiling expression of a dissociated person in such condition, and asks me if I know what spirit he is. Since I know he often represents the spirit of a young man of high rank who was drowned at sea thirty years before, I say "Yes." He says "You know they call me Satan (he means the Christian missionaries). But I am one who was lost at sea, and who comes to help the sick." Then he asks my view of his proceedings and again stresses that anything he does is only for good ends. After urging the patient to eat again, and prescribing hot application, discussing the symptoms with the girl's father and other kin, the spirit announces his departure. With flapping, quivering movements of the hands, almost in dance-form, the state of dissociation ends.

The next day we go again. The practitioner emphasizes that not a day must pass without a visit to his patient—a sick person gets constant attention. When we get to the house a bowl of hot water is prepared, by making a special magical stone red-hot on the fire and plunging it into the vessel of liquid. With this hot water the back and side of the patient are bathed. The practitioner gets a girl to fill her mouth with water and squirt it over his hands while he washes them, and he himself takes a drink and cleanses his mouth by squirting water out of the door. Then he again enters a state of dissociation, and continues the massage and other treatment as before. There is an animated discussion of the cause of the illness and its prognosis. Finally the practitioner says to his patient "Now it has gone; it is over."

Indeed, the patient by this time is feeling much better. This is not surprising, because she has also been visited twice by the medical dresser. He says that her temperature last night was 104°F., that he gave her drugs, and that today her temperature has fallen to 99°F.

This case illustrates several primitive notions about health and disease. First, the cause of the illness—we diagnosed it as an influenzal infection, probably with pleurisy. The local practitioner said it was due to an evil spirit. This spirit, dwelling in a rock near the seashore, had objected, he said, to the girl's father having built a house nearby, and had made the girl sick in consequence. Secondly, the illness was interpreted as the result of a breach

—a mistake in siting the house—not by the patient herself but by her father. Sickness often is looked upon as suffering for someone else's errors. It is a form of indirect retribution. Looking at the matter more empirically, the anthropologist sees this as an expression of some disapproval or doubt by the practitioner himself. Unconsciously, perhaps, the spirit-healer really thinks the house was put in the wrong place. In other words, the physical phenomenon of illness gives an occasion for a social judgment. Diagnosis is a symbolic way of giving an outlet to some social problem or opinion. Thirdly, the treatment by the local spirit-medium practitioner was only of marginal value. He had his own ideas of cleanliness, but they did not conform to modern scientific ideas of hygiene. His massage may have been harmless, and his hot water application soothing, but they were purely external alleviation; these people have no internal remedies of any value. The patient's speedy recovery in this case must be attributed primarily to the medicines of the Western-trained dresser, although the people gave most of the credit to the spirit-healer.

We ask then, why, as soon as the services of such a Western-trained man become available, do not the people drop their local quacks, and simply follow the new treatment?

I have hinted at some of the reasons already. Treatment of the sick in such communities is a highly social matter. Relatives, friends, neighbors assemble. Even if they just sit around, their presence helps to cheer the invalid, to reassure her that she is not isolated from her society, to make her feel a focus of interest. They cannot simply abandon her to foreign care. Then, the theory of this illness, like many other, involves spiritual as well as physical causation. Consequently it involves spiritual as well as physical therapy. It gives a very important psychological reassurance to patient and relatives. Moreover, the practitioners have a strong vested interest in using traditional diagnosis to get expression for social judgment. They use diagnosis—as the Manus of New Guinea do—to express a moral attitude or to bolster up a factional interest. They use spirit verdicts to add weight to this. All this is built up into an elaborate system of beliefs and practices which a foreign medical man is not expected to use or understand, but in proof of which many successful cases are cited. Moreover, the people believe this system to be more profound. Hence they do not abandon their own practitioners who know, they believe, how to handle these elaborate, often malevolent spirit powers.

Yet this community is quite receptive to new ideas. There is no opposition to new medical treatment, though some timidity may have to be overcome with a person faced with drugs or inoculation. There is a rough dichotomy of illness and infirmity into those afflictions which come "of themselves," that is, naturally, and those more severe or refractory ones which are caused by spirit agency. But Western medicines are welcomed for the latter as for the former; the people have rearranged their concepts of health and disease to admit the use of a whole range of non-traditional therapeutic agents. Moerover, the local practitioners, spirit-mediums or "medicine men," are likewise not antipathetic to the new therapy. They are happy to intermingle their own simple systems of leaf infusions, massage, and prayerful laying on of hands with the administration of Western pills. These practitioners are almost pathetically anxious to gain Western approval. They are convinced that their spirit techniques are correct, but are under fire from modernists in their own community.

Medicine has become a weapon in a factional struggle. So the spirit-healers emphasize the morality of their task. Their healing art is a good art, they say.

It will be clear now that in a community of this sort, in the diagnosis of an illness and treatment of the patient, one is working not merely at the physical level; very important mental components, both intellectual and emotional, are also involved. Moreover, the patient is not an individual to be treated singly and alone; he lives in a social context, and one which has a moral tone. Understanding of concepts of health and disease, of actions related to them, and of the way they change, necessitates a knowledge of the social system with its structure, its cleavages, its factions, its loyalties and associated values, including moral values.

What I have described from this fairly simple Polynesian community I could have analysed in greater detail from a more sophisticated community I studied in Malaya, and paralleled from the studies of other anthropologists in many parts of the world. It is primarily this social character of ideas of health and disease, the way in which they are interrelated with other ideas and with patterns of behavior in a community, which results in traditional concepts being retained so long in the face of much modernization in other ways.

For example, look for a moment at the position of the Maori of New Zealand, among whom acculturation has gone a very long way indeed. The Maori people have provided the country with doctors, lawyers, Members of Parliament and others of high distinction. Such men are Western in their outlook on medicine. Yet among many Maoris some traditional concepts of health and disease also still persist. Old taboos often operate. One is that things associated with cooked food at some stages are contaminating to a person. So it is still not uncommon in rural Maori homes to find a rigid separation between receptacles used for preparing food or washing up cooking utensils and dishes, and basins used to wash the hands and face. The towel for dishes must never touch the head, and neither hands nor body may be washed in the kitchen sink. The country New Zealander of European descent is much less careful, and even the baby is often bathed in the kitchen sink. This is horrifying to many Maori mothers. Illness or even death is believed to be caused by such breach of taboo. So some Maoris carry over their ancient ritual taboo into the field of health.

Concepts of sorcery and evil spirits also exist among some Maori communities, influencing their concepts of disease and their attitudes toward medical aid. The *tohunga,* the Maori expert in medico-magical skills, still exists, though he has modernized his techniques. Most of the activities of such a man are harmless, concerned with herbal remedies and the like, but some dabble in the manipulation of spirits.

Recently, a six-year old Maori child was believed to harbor an evil spirit. On the recommendation of an expert he was regularly dipped in cold water at dawn and sunset through summer and winter; alternately, he was shut in a room and beaten, to drive out the spirit. Some of this treatment was performed by the child's mother, at the instance of the expert. The father disapproved of such practices. He finally called public attention to them by firing rifle bullets through the expert's house at a range of about one hundred yards. When he was charged with this offense, the (*pakeha*) Court appreciated his motive and admitted him on probation for good behavior without punishment.[2]

In some Maori communities, again, there is an aversion to Western medicine. Maori women sometimes refuse to accept hospitalization, maternity home or sanitarium treatment. They will not leave the community. The reason for this may be partly fear of being isolated from family and neighbors, of being removed from the social unit. It may also be due partly to ideas that hospital hygiene is different from Maori hygiene, and that one may get one's face washed in a basin that has been in the kitchen. When Maori mothers go to maternity homes—as they do in large numbers—some of the more conservative ones still have the traditional taboos relating to childbirth removed from mother and baby before they venture to return home—a kind of absolution ritual. This allows them formally to be reintegrated into their community. In some cases, resistance to modern medical treatment is due to the influence of a *tohunga* who feels that his status and livelihood are threatened by Westernized competition.

Much of what I have said about the Maori of New Zealand could be paralleled by instances from the Navaho, the Zuni, the Papago and other Indian communities of the United States, who in many respects are in a similar situation in this country to the Maori in New Zealand. To both peoples over two centuries, acculturation has brought, alongside great material benefits, disease and decimation and political embarrassment. Their growing confidence in Western medicine has thus been an act of political faith as well as an alteration in health concepts and treatment.

[2] J. Phillipps (13) pp. 179-181; articles on Tohunga cults in *New Zealand Herald,* April 3 and Oct. 19, 1955.

This analysis is applicable not merely to remote, primitive or small-scale populations. Resistance to new ideas constitutes one of the basic medical problems in many parts of the world—even our own. Ignorance, stupidity and fear play their part in such attitudes. But the situation is much more complex, being governed by an intricate set of cultural relations and values in each society. This makes for change along some lines and obduracy along others. As the work of anthropologists has demonstrated, in Central and South America, India, Indonesia, Africa and New Guinea, medicine, including concepts of health and disease, must be looked upon as part of a social and cultural system.[3] The degree to which it is integrated with other parts of the system, however, may differ considerably. To mark a broad contrast, in Western society medicine is more closely linked with technology than with religion, while for a traditional oriental society the reverse is apt to be the case. But even in the West certain religious bodies have their own special official attitudes toward medicine or toward some medical practices. No department of the healing art, even surgery, can claim to be an entirely independent variable.

Hence in seeking relations between acculturation and concepts of health and disease, we cannot look at purely medical innovations alone. Indeed, it is a pertinent question to ask whether the most important changes in the health field may not come from influences outside the medical sphere. It is tempting to suggest that for many of the underdeveloped areas of the world really major

[3] Mention can be made here of studies by only a few, e.g.: George M. Foster, Richard N. Adams, Benjamin D. Paul, Ozzie C. Simmons, Lyle Saunders, Maurice Freedman and his wife Judith Djamour, Isabel Kelly, Edward Wellin, R. N. Rapoport, G. M. Carstairs, McKim Marriott, Margaret McArthur.

advances in health will come only with a significant rise in the level of per capita income. Medicine, it may be argued, is a signpost, not a vehicle along the road of progress. It takes advantage of a favorable economic climate to indicate ways in which standards of comfort may be raised.

Concepts of health are basically altered only by radical changes in the content and structure of economic and social life. To put the issue only like this would of course be grossly unfair. We have only to think for a moment of the work of men like Lister on antisepsis, of Laveran, Grassi, Ross and Watson on malaria, of Noguchi, Stokes and others on yellow fever, to realize how the ideas of people about the maintenance of their health can be rapidly changed by the development of medical knowledge as such. Moreover, medical developments may facilitate economic developments, as malaria control has enabled men to work in safety agricultural land which previously had to lie waste. But the task lies as much in implementation as in discovery. Such medical developments can take place only in a favorable social and economic milieu—as the scientific developments of Vesalius and others in anatomy in the 16th century were aided by the fresh viewpoint and interest of the painter and sculptor in the human body. It is in this sense that the extramedical factors may be so important, for the reasons, in general, which lead people in a society to alter their attitudes to health and disease may come from extramedical stimuli and opportunities—including those in the economic sphere.

But before turning to examine this theme, I want to look at the concepts of health and disease again, more closely, and from a comparative point of view. Definitions of health are legion. At one end of the scale you have the joking definition of a healthy man as one who takes stairs two at a time and not pills two at a time. This is the practical man's notion, the attractive male image of the perpetually young, athletic type. It ignores the disagreeable reminders of advancing age with its arterial complications. Like many other popular definitions of health, it is concerned with limited specific physical norms.

Very different are the concepts of health of those whose profession it is to think about the subject in a broad way. I have referred already to the World Health Organization's definition. Health as a state of complete physical, mental and social well-being is not a norm, but an optimum. As a goal a modern international organization can point to no less. It is a part of the common discontent with things as they are—and as they will continue to be—which helps to give meaning to human activity.

Such an all-embracing definition has its difficulties. There is the practical question of what objectives should actually be aimed at in any given period, considering the limitations on resources both in finance and personnel in any field situation. Again, what indices do we use to measure well-being? Granted, that for the physical and mental aspects we can find some acceptable measures, but what about health as a state of *social* well-being?—political freedom, the opportunity to realize innate endowments, provision for satisfaction of aesthetic and emotional capacities, and so on, I suppose. But how do we measure these conditions? Historically, and even nowadays, large sections of world society will almost certainly disagree as to how far these conditions were and are being fulfilled in their own countries. There is still another question. Physical and mental well-being are related to social well-being, but may not coincide with it. A well-nourished body and a free mind do not always go together. Social well-being is normally a precondition of mental and physical well-being, but they should not be confused.

On the other hand, a little reflection makes it clear that to define health simply in terms of external physical conditions is not enough. To be able to take stairs two at a time may rejoice the mind of a man—but what about the strain on his heart? Moreover it has a hint of that sense of urgency which is so much a part of our industrial and urban life, and of which part of the effects emerge in what has been called the stress syndrome. This sacrifice of the physical to the mental through the pressure of interest, ambition and obligation is not new. In the year of the French Revolution, Arthur Young, touring in France, noted one morning that he woke up with a sore throat. He attributed his feverishness to the heat. His diary continued: "I was inclined to waste a day here for the security of my health; but we are all fools in trifling with the things most valuable to us. Loss of time and vain expense are always in the head of a man who travels as much as I am forced to do." But in this case his energy was more soundly based than his fears. He covered twenty-two miles that day, and twenty-seven the next, without ill effect (20, p. 85).

In all cultural systems studied by anthropologists, concepts of health assume some kind of integral condition of the human personality, with a functioning that it is improper to disturb. In the Western field, etymology itself often indicates this: *health* and *Heilung* are related to the idea of wholeness; *santé, sanitá,* and the basic Latin *sanus* link the notion of health with avoidance of disintegrating effects of extremes; *malady* and its congeners relate to the notion of bad arrangement. In non-Western systems the terms are often more specific, but similar ideas are involved. One Malay expression for health is *sĕdap badan,* ease of body. And of the Indians of Yucatan it is stated "Health of body and peace of soul depend upon the maintenance of conditions of balance. Extremes and the meeting of extremes are to be avoided" (15, p. 128). But while in very general terms these concepts are analogous to those of the West, the precise kind of integrity or balance envisaged is often very different. In popular Muslim ideology the wholeness of the body is important in a very literal sense, so that surgical operations which might involve amputation, for example, are looked upon with repugnance. Then again, the integrity of the body is regarded in many cultural systems as depending fundamentally upon the integrity of some vital or spiritual essence of the personality which we may briefly call the soul. If the soul is damaged, the body becomes sick.

Hence illness indicates a weakness not in the bodily defenses but in the spiritual defenses. This may sometimes be due to simple passivity of the personality, its openness to attack, as when a child becomes ill because it has been attacked by evil spirits. Or it may be due to some wrong act of the person, a breach of taboo, an adulterous relationship, a failure to make ritual offerings or to recite due prayers for the dead.

Implications from this are first that defense against illness and disease demands watchfulness on the part of responsible persons to see that members of their family and their community are not in a vulnerable state. This may mean prayer, religious austerity and the like. It usually also means a category of specialists charged with protective functions. Secondly, illness may be itself a moral condemnation, and a proof of moral delinquency. Hence people in some cultures could agree with Samuel Butler's Erewhonians that the sick should be put in gaol, not in hospitals. Thirdly, a considerable part of the energies of a healer may have to go into warding off the *spiritual* forces opposed to the patient. He may have to restore the patient's personal and psychological equilibrium, not merely his bodily equilibrium, as a precedent to restoring bodily health. Fourthly, such a medicine man, shaman, *curandero,* etc., is not a charlatan. He is to his people a doughty fighter in the cause of health, and for them one who is more profound in his search for causes, more likely to destroy the roots of disease in a person than the Western-trained doctor who treats only the bodily symptoms.

This may sound to us a surrealist kind of medicine—or just plain nonsense. But what these people have been seeking is a double kind of expression. First, they have sought some form of analogy, some way of rendering in words the concepts of these largely invisible, intangible phenomena which we call health and disease. As Snouck Hurgronje (8, vol. I, p. 409) wrote of the Achehnese fifty years ago, they talk not of microbes but of spirits which threaten man with all manner of evils. Why then cannot they be easily induced to think of microbes instead of spirits when new medical knowledge is brought to them? Because, in their theory of health and disease, they also try to account for selectivity. Why do the microbes affect one person and not another, they ask; and answer, because the microbes are directed by spirits, who pick and choose the objects of their ill will.

So the second aspect of these concepts is a theory of incidence. They give a volitional character to what we know as the random effects of microagents of disease. They translate the disease agencies from some impersonal element into a personal, motivated entity, the spirit. In this way disease is brought, as it were, within the compass of action. One can do something about personal beings, one can make them retreat, or one can thwart their aims. Again, there is an element of purpose, or intention, attributed. The disease is represented not as the blind striking of fate, but of some purposive act on the part of a spirit —often stimulated thereto, indeed, by some other human being, out of malice. Here the theory of incidence has seen, however dimly, that there is some relation between man's physical well-being and his social circumstances— though for the most part they have misconceived the nature of this relation. They have attributed to aggression, frustration, malice and uncharitableness a positive direct power over human health instead of a negative, indirect power.

But our inferences from all this must be, first, that such a system can be completely intelligible to us—though it has a different frame. And secondly, the close link of the physical with the psychosocial elements in the system means that it is unlikely to yield easily to a straightforward medical assault—unless of a very sophisticated kind.

Here is a suggestion of the very popular word, "psychosomatic." From one point of view there is much in common between folk concepts of health and Western concepts in their recognition of the relation between mind and body in illness. But a significant difference is seen between most Western and non-Western situations. In the West a psychosomatic illness is one in which the patient expresses bodily disease (lack of ease in a literal sense), some psychological condition of strain or maladjustment. The illness is a personal expression or symbolization of this strain or conflict. It is also up to a point a solution of the conflict, as a short-term measure. The patient escapes from his immediate obligation by taking to bed, running a temperature, and so on. By the diagnostic physician there is established a direct, if often vague, relation between the psychological condition and the physical condition, so that if the former be altered the illness may disappear. To this extent there may be public skepticism about the "reality" of the illness. That is, patient, physician and public may have divergent views about its independent status, about the relations involved, and about the treatment.

Usually, in folk medicine the situation is almost in reverse. In non-Western situations there are some psychosomatic illnesses too—though not usually overtly recognized as such by the society. An illness may be regarded as a symbol of psychological conditions of strain, family conflict, etc., and indeed a direct expression of such through witchcraft or sorcery. The local diagnostic physician, medicine man, etc., makes an identification between the psychosocial condition and the physical condition. Hence he alters the psychological or spiritual condition in order to alter the illness and make it disappear. But the symbolism expressed in the illness is socially shared. There is full, or fairly full, agreement among patient, physician and public, though some disagreement may arise over the attribution of precise cause in terms of the person responsible. Moreover to the external, Western-trained observer, the illness usually *has* an independent status. There are parallel, not linked, phenomena in the mental-physical field. And yet the therapy may be reminiscent. To the Western view the local curative attempts on most of these diseases are almost bound to fail. Yet to the non-Western view the Western cures may seem to have only superficial success. If the underlying strains, tensions, breach of rules have not been cleared up, the people—and the patient—may remain unconvinced that there will be an effective and lasting recovery. It is true that Western therapy has made great strides in the non-Western world. But it is not true that such curative measures are always their own advertisement. A wider alteration of the belief system may be necessary for their effectiveness to be demonstrated to the satisfaction of the local people.

The facts of resistance are well known; they have been amply documented by health workers and anthropologists. It has often been pointed out that what seem to be ignorance and stupidity may be just reticence and timidity. But the resistance often goes far deeper. One kind of block against effective therapy is what may be termed the witchcraft block. In Afghanistan and Vietnam, the taking of blood samples for antivenereal and other campaigns was resisted because it was thought that the blood might be used to deliver the personality of the owner into the hands of an enemy. In Northern Australia the taking of stools samples for study of intestinal parasites was resisted for an analogous reason.

More commonly, however, the block arises within the more general structure of the local health frame. There is a prejudice against hospitals and maternity centers, because, as in Quito (Ecuador), the fresh air of a hospital is bad for women in childbirth, or among the Maoris there may be contamination with cooked food, or in Kelantan (rural Malaya), a hospital is a place for "cutting," which is repugnant to any good Muslim. Very widely, too, it is believed that a hospital is a place where only dying people go.[4] There may also be a prejudice against certain foods. In Vietnam, cows' milk is considered repugnant, and in Western Nigeria, while there is no taboo upon it, there is a widespread conviction that it is only needed to puff up European children, who would die if they did not get it. In Micronesia some traditional beliefs about infant feeding are still believed: in Ponape raw fish, mangoes, or pineapples eaten by a lactating mother are thought to cause prickly heat in the infant; in Palau it is held that taro gives yaws to infants and that they should not have fish or eggs in their first year (11, pp. 8, 15). In Kelantan (Malaya) even the father is involved; the husband of a pregnant woman is forbidden to eat certain kinds of fish lest the child be harmed.

Disease again may be regarded as "natural." Smallpox, in many Asiatic countries, has been looked upon as sent by the gods, a necessity for man to endure. Yaws, in the South Pacific, has been regarded as a disease which it is good to get over in childhood. And to Dr. Anne Burgess I am indebted for the illustration of a Malay grandmother, who on one occasion squashed all the doctor's arguments about a child by saying firmly, "But a Malay child *must* have worms, Mem!"

In these and many other ways the programs of curative and preventive medicine are impeded, owing to lack of agreement on concepts of health and disease between practitioners and people. But in the societies with which we are dealing there are other and perhaps more important reasons. The hospital to the sick person is an alien

[4] The hospital regarded as "the place where people die" is reminiscent of the attitude of James Young Simpson and others in Europe a hundred years ago. Before the discoveries of Semmelweiss and Lister, forty per cent of the admissions to hospitals died of sepsis and other infections, and the case for abandonment of "hospitalism" was strongly made accordingly.

place. It is unlike his home, and he often gets food very different from that to which he is used. He is often deprived of the care of his kin, and conversely they have no opportunity to perform for him the obligations which are regarded as their due. Hence the whole concept of being hospitalized is something antipathetic and frightening.

In 1945 I visited a leper hospital on the Nigerian Plateau. There had been great difficulty in persuading the shy pagans of the plateau to come for hospital treatment in the stark bare wards, away from their home and relatives. But the mission doctor in charge evolved a method to overcome their resistance. Their own houses are small and round, with tiny doorways and no windows, dark and warm inside. He built his hospital wards as small rooms, allowed them to be filled with grassy beds to which the people were accustomed, and let the patients have their families around. They flocked for treatment, and he was also able to keep an eye on their kinsfolk, to see if signs of the disease should develop in them too.

Like most other social anthropologists, I am interested in change as much as in the traditional and resistant. Many changes have been recorded in the direction of acceptance of new therapy. In Navaho land the tuberculosis hospitals are full; Navaho women prefer to have their babies in maternity hospitals. The Makah Indians of the North West summon a doctor by telephone and let a patient be flown off to the hospital in an airplane. When Redfield (15) was in Chan Kom in 1931, only one man used store-bought medicines and hypodermic injections. By 1948 such remedies were generally known and widely used. Several young women had been taught to use the hypodermic syringe, and there was knowledge of penicillin which several of the villagers had had administered to them in the city. One of the most marked acceptances of alien methods has been that of injection. In Formosa and right down throughout the South Pacific the value of this treatment for yaws and other conditions has long been recognized (4, p. 100). Among the Navaho, traditionally resistant to foreign medicine, it is common for a person to bring along a child for injection, saying "Baby sick. You give shot." Among the Yoruba it has been said that the most acceptable part of Western treatment is undoubtedly the hypodermic needle, in the power of which there is almost blind faith. Among many people there it is considered almost as a magical instrument, exerting its power over disease like a charm.

How do such changes take place, and what is their distribution?

The first thing to note is that people in all societies with backward medical practice and unscientific concepts of disease do sooner or later learn some things by experience. It has been very widely recorded how even local lay practitioners of the traditional "medicine man" type enthusiastically add the simpler Western drugs of obvious curative effect to their pharmacopeia. Aspirin and its allies *do* relieve pain and fever; quinine and the associated antimalarial drugs are often used, sometimes together with local herbal remedies. They, like injections, may be regarded as panaceas for a range of ailments far wider than those with which they actually cope. In other words, they may come to have a quasi-magical value.

Secondly, people can learn to revise their concepts by the need to conform to some wide-scale organizational action. For example, the institution of a protected water supply and the provision of large numbers of cheap shoes may help people to alter very considerably their notions about the origination of dysentery and hookworm. But mass solutions of this latter kind are not always easy and are very limited in number. If, for example, another organizational "automatic" type of public health service is provided in the form of sanitary privies, the effect may be somewhat different. In the first case, if the people use water at all they may be bound to use the protected supply—the alternative may be almost impossible for them. But in the case of new sanitary arrangements, particularly in rural areas, the old alternatives of using the bushes may be simpler than the new arrangement, or at least, as easy. The problem here then is not merely to *institute* the new technology; it is to ensure that people *utilize* it. There are a number of cases on record where such new sanitary arrangements either have not been utilized or required some local adaptation to make them fit the notions of the people as to the way in which their processes of elimination should be properly carried out. We have, for instance, by now the almost classic case of the sanitary privies from which the roofs had to be removed in order that people might have the sensation, traditional to them, of easing themselves under the shade of trees, in the open air (6, p. 13).

Any change in concepts of health and disease may be assisted then by linking what is desired with some existing practices and concepts of the people. This is exemplified in another way by the possibility of linking new medical treatment with the work of the local practitioners of traditional style. In Costa Rica, for example, the popularity of such lay practitioners as *curanderos,* midwives and pharmacists lies, it is said, in the ability of these people to play the doctor role to such an extent as to overshadow their technical deficiencies. By this is meant that they are in intimate contact with the members of the community and are often in a position to find in the network of social relationships factors related to psychosomatic illness. Therefore at times they can actually cure patients with such illnesses when a physician of modern type may find himself unable to do so. Again, not merely illness but also problems of a moral order may be referred to them—rather as the old-fashioned general practitioner was often made the confidant of his patients on non-medical matters. When to these various aspects of the doctor's role is added the fact that their services may often be less expensive than those of a Western-trained medical man, one can realize how they maintain their position in the community. The inference from this is that if the cooperation of these lay medical practitioners can be enlisted, if informal relations of a friendly kind can be established with them, then the improvement of sanitary and health practices can proceed at a much more rapid pace.

This fits the general proposition, often put forward by anthropologists and others, that if education, medical or other developmental processes are to contribute effectively, then they should be latched on to existing beliefs and practices wherever possible. In such conditions, Loomis and others argue, "A knowledge of existing beliefs and practices is invaluable, and the teacher or extension agent, who understands these systems, is in a better position to broaden his work and make it more efficient" (10, pp. 135, 147-148).

While in general I think this is very true, such a proposition may be only one step towards a solution. There are three difficult questions to solve. The first is: just what are the existing beliefs and practices which it is necessary to take account of (and by contrast, those which can be ignored or should be combated)? It is often said nowadays that a medical man should learn "something" about the customs and beliefs of the people among whom he is going to work. But *what* precisely does he need to learn? An unsystematic collection of scraps of information may lead to an exaggerated respect for taboos and an underestimation of the importance of features of the society which may throw a medical program out of gear. The second question is, granted that this knowledge has been ascertained, how is it to be integrated effectively into any program of medical training, at what stage, and by whom? And the third question is, granted the requisite local knowledge has been obtained and supplied to the medical profession, what does the doctor do about it?—what decisions does he make on the spot, if local beliefs and treatment are in direct contradiction to good medical practices?

There are no easy answers to these questions, but I am sure that the road to finding answers lies not in turning our backs upon the problems but in gaining more knowledge about them. In this field, the delicate and sensitive sphere of interpersonal relations, there are few spectacular discoveries to be made. But even to understand the major issues and the social background is an advance.

It is increasingly clear, for instance, that changes in health and disease concepts are frequently uneven for any given society, and may produce results unexpected by the Western practitioner. Consider nutrition. In the earlier days of tropical medicine, major efforts were directed toward the reduction of parasitic complaints, such as malaria or the helminthic disorders, and of infectious diseases, while nutritional needs tended to be overlooked. In recent years the emphasis has changed. The urge to see that diets are improved wherever possible by better provision of proteins and vitamins has produced its effect. In a number of Latin-American countries the notion of vitamins has penetrated, with the idea that they are important for nutrition. But this has been very uneven. In Turrialba (Costa Rica) about half the persons interviewed had heard of vitamins and their nutritional role. But their nutritional knowledge in other directions was much more scanty, and not fitted into their everyday behavior. Four fifths of them said they would not be willing to accept skim milk, either fluid or dried, and most believed it had little food value. Of the mothers interviewed, two fifths had lost all their teeth through faulty diet. In the community as a whole good diets seemed generally to be related to purchasing power and to home farm production, rather than to any superior nutritional knowledge as such (10, pp. 137, 143).[5] In Ica (Peru) there is a crude notion of *vitaminas*. But the idea is that good or beneficial foods have many vitamins, and that most vitamin foods are fattening and body-building. Moreover, it is believed that vitamins A, B, C, etc., are of descending value according to their order in the alphabet.[6] Such concepts raise the question of whether what may be termed "provitaminosis" is necessarily better than avitaminosis.

What effect have these changes had upon the general system of health and disease ideas? For many of the so-called underdeveloped countries it would seem that changes in diet and the acceptance of a new therapy have not so much altered the traditional conceptions of health and disease as produced additions to them. As Redfield

[5] This is an inference from the data there given, not a direct quotation.

[6] My colleague Maurice Freedman has told me that in many parts of Indonesia the word *fitamin* or *pitamin* is used, sometimes jocularly, sometimes seriously, to describe simply excellence in food.

has reported for Chan Kom, while there were many changes in therapy, conceptions as to the *causes* of sickness appear in many cases to remain much as they were. He points out that although in 1931 some instruction in the germ theory of disease was given to the people of Chan Kom, and though the Cultural Mission of 1944/45 strove to improve the understanding of the people in regard to scientific ideas of health and hygiene, on his visit there in 1948 he heard nothing from the people about microbes and infections. A suggestion that the common cold passes by contagion was met by expressions of amusement. This is a very general situation.

Where a medicine man or other lay practitioner has accepted modern drugs he may use them or ask for them to be administered by a Western person as a preliminary or accompaniment to his own spiritual ministrations. I cited one case of this from the South Pacific. I remember, too, a medicine man in Malaya who was due to come to my house one evening and conduct a spirit-medium performance to cure a sick person. Shortly before he was due, a messenger arrived saying that he could not come. He was ill himself with fever. He demanded the usual anti-malarial drugs, which of course I sent him. When we discussed it on his recovery, he saw no inconsistency. His fever was a perfectly natural illness which could be cured by Western drugs. The illness he was coming to cure had been caused by spirits whom no Western medicines could touch. Yet this was fifty years after Western medicine had been in operation in that Malay area. Moreover, drugs are often acceptable when more elaborate forms of treatment are not. In Malaya and Java, for example, anthropologists have found an eager desire for drugs, especially when administered by people whom the local folk knew well, but an indifference or hostility to the general system of Western medicine of which the drugs are really a part.

Folk conceptions of health and disease are, then, by no means rigid. They have a flexibility which can absorb new ways and new ideas. But the result is on the whole to *enlarge* the scope of their therapy rather than radically to *overthrow* the framework of their health ideology.

There are also more subtle and more complex results. The traditional system of folk medicine tends to be homogeneous, fairly evenly distributed through the community as far as belief in it is concerned. Specialist practitioners have, of course, their own secrets and techniques of skill. But both they and their patients share the same general framework of ideas in regard to the exercise of those secrets and skills. With the persistent pressure of Western medical concepts, some heterogeneity is usually introduced. Local nurses, hospital attendants and doctors are trained in Western methods and inevitably their conceptual framework in handling their practical problems does alter. An African doctor from Nigeria or Uganda may share with his Western colleagues the same framework of scientific medicine so fully that he is more strongly opposed even than they to the traditional folk medicine. Attempts to justify it or compromise with it in the interests of good social relations he may regard as surrender to the forces of ignorance and wrong thinking. The existence of such men, devoted to the ideals of Western scientific medical practice marks a split in the society, a contrast with other sections who still uphold traditional conceptions. This is not just a medical situation. Medical development creates new social structures. This unevenness of change may in itself produce conflict in a society and inhibit medical work.

In these other sections of society, the influences of

change may also have been at work. The possibility of alternative treatments as between Western and traditional style, while it widens the field of therapy, may also lead to uncertainty. People may become confused as to where truth lies when, as often happens, the Western and the indigenous practitioner give diametrically opposite advice. As Redfield has pointed out for Chan Kom, people nowadays in such conditions are less easily resigned to die, while they are more troubled about how to live. A sickness has a more varied and less self-consistent course than formerly, when the medicine man was the sole source of appeal. The lack of a coherent system of medical knowledge and belief is one of the difficulties that is likely to be encountered as Western medicine penetrates more deeply into the fabric of local institutions. Moreover, Western medical ideas and treatment do not advance alone. With them come the whole panoply of Western consumer goods and new wants associated with them.

Attitudes toward the use of milk illustrate both the possibilities of change and its effects. In some cases the change has been quite rapid. About 1930, adults in the Gilbert Islands did not like canned milk, and could not understand the white man's liking for milk in puddings and other foods. All food of this class they said was " a thing to make vomit." By about 1949 milk had come into use. Though on medical recommendation the greater proportion of it was bought for their children, the adults themselves had developed a taste for it, and added it to their diet when money permitted (18, p. 43). But in Uganda, things have gone differently. On the one hand there has been complaint that large cattle-keeping populations drink little milk (e.g., the Lango). But where the production of milk has been stimulated under European tutelage, it is not always consumed by the people themselves, but is diverted to earn an income. In fact the Uganda Nutrition Committee reports rather sadly that in and around the larger towns with a large European population, there is already proof that the monetary return for marketing is acting as a deterrent to home consumption of milk by the small peasant producer and his family. The solution of the African nutritional problem then, it was admitted, is not quite so easy (19, p. 11).

The same holds true for stimulation of meat production. In the East African area, while all tribes eat meat occasionally, it has not been a regular item of diet in quantity with some of them. In prewar days the African often did not want to sell his stock, partly because of relative scarcity, owing to the toll taken by epizootic and endemic diseases, and partly because of the symbolic value attached to them. But with improved disease control and Westernization, African stock owners began to take advantage of the market, and also improved their cattle. The steady development in the number of cattle sold and slaughtered for the many meat markets has meant that a meat ration has become a regular part of the native diet in many areas. But while the Uganda Nutrition Committee notes that the Government's efforts to stimulate meat consumption have met with considerable success, it also finds that "unfortunately, progress has been so rapid that a state has now been reached when consumption exceeds replacements" (19). In other words, the value of a foodstuff for nutrition may be largely determined by its position in the budget and resources of the people. A particular foodstuff may be withdrawn from their diet by a competing price attraction, or put back by means of income from some other source. It is often the economic situation, then, rather than medical action as such, which dictates a change in food habits.

This, of course, comes as no surprise to us. In the West, it is well known that factors outside the medical sphere have historically been responsible for medical changes. For example, the causes of improvement in the sanitation of London in the eighteenth century were only partly those of conscious effort in street clearing. One factor of note was the influence of improved agriculture—it created a demand for the filth of the streets for manure for the rural land (7, p. 55). Again, we are familiar with the arguments about the breast-feeding of infants. Some of us may know of the fierce addiction to formula-feeding shown by some immigrant mothers in the United States, wanting to become true Americans. By contrast it is interesting to note that Arthur Young remarked in 1787 that women of the first fashion in France had by then become ashamed of not nursing their own children. He attributed this largely to the enlightening influence of the ideas spread by Jean Jacques Rousseau. Be this as it may, it is certainly not simply the perception of the value of mother's milk, but a complex of social factors—including status or prestige factors—which have determined in many different states of society the pendulum swing between breast-feeding and "formula"-feeding for infants.

Acculturation is not an unmixed blessing for health. The medical problem then may increasingly come to be not one of persuading people to abandon the old in favor of the new, but of restraining them from selecting those features in the new which are medically of no more value or even less value than the old. It is reported that some Eskimos nowadays will buy canned peaches when they need canned milk. Among the Sotho of South Africa (2,

p. 19) the use of refined maize meal and flour is growing and supplanting the use of home-ground wholemeal flour. The new-bought refined products are ready to cook and so encourage many people to buy them during weeding and harvest. Moreover they save women labor and time in grinding their grain, in addition to their ordinary agricultural tasks. Many Sotho dislike these refined meals and say that they have less body and substance than the wholemeal flour. Medically there may be something to be said for this view. The incidence of pellagra has been tentatively ascribed to the use of milled maize. Yet time saving, ostentation and taste all prompt their use.

The medical man here is up against a similar problem to that which faces him in our own Western countries in the use of bread. This "staff of life" has been so vitaminized, fortified, improved, preserved and aerated that the original balance of its nutritional qualities and perhaps even its value as a nutritional mainstay, is very much in doubt. Nowadays, man certainly cannot live by bread alone.

From this several inferences may be drawn. It is clear that the most successful type of health measure may well be that which can be made effective in the mass, without calling upon the intellectual agreement of the people to any radical degree. As Scheele has pointed out (17, p. 19), some of the most dramatic results have come from applying controls to the physical environment, as for example, where a safe water supply has been established without even the knowledge of many individuals, millions of whom have been protected against intestinal infections without ever realizing what was happening. Likewise with inoculations, in which only the acquiescence of the patient is needed, not his understanding. But where an active cooperation, not merely a passive acquiescence, is required the task is much more difficult. Not only may there be vested interests to encounter, but more and more, as the gross medical problems are being met, the tendency is for responsibility for the maintenance of personal health to rest on the individual himself. Exercise, rest, diet, alcohol intake, reporting of illness, avoidance of contagion require in the last resort, for adults at least, a personal care and a personal decision. The problem here is how to condition the individual to take medical care of himself. In the long run a vast amount of health work must take place in the home. It is in the home, as health educators well realize, that the implementation of most new ideas is ultimately required. Here is the test of new concepts. And here is apt to be the most refractory field of operation. Wellin's example of water boiling is revealing here. In a Peruvian village a very competent health visitor energetically tried for over two years to persuade housewives to boil their contaminated drinking water. Out of two hundred households, fifteen were already boiling their water when she arrived, and she was able to add only eleven more to the list—an additional six per cent. The complex conceptions, economic, social and ritual, which entered into this baffling situation may be more elaborate than in many other cases of home health measures, but in general they illustrate the major difficulty.

This example draws attention to several implications of health education. One is that education, to be effective, should probably be general and not specific. It is in raising the general educational level, not merely in promoting specific health ideas, that advance may have to come. Again, changes in concepts of health and disease very often seem to be in response to the devoted efforts of men and women who work within a relatively small radius. It is upon people who know and trust them that their effect operates. How is one to get scale into such operations? This may have to be a long-term effect; there are few shortcuts. It is often said that the local person is too susceptible to the local standards of etiquette, achievement and status to push his community beyond the level at which they are satisfied. Yet surely the only way to get a health program accepted in the end is to have trained local people in whom their fellows will have confidence. Often this policy has borne remarkable fruit (5). But there is no automatic answer here; only experiment, and sociological sensitivity can tell.

These questions of scale of work, relation of medical personnel to the local community, length of time to achieve results, degree of association with general education, are all becoming more relevant with the change in the medical and public health field itself. In the West, as is well known, the control of physical environment, and the diagnosis and treatment of infectious diseases and immunization against them have been tackled with great success. The task, it is realized, has now begun to change in emphasis to the fields of chronic disease, mental disease and lowered physical tone. Effort is now directed to more individual problems, and programs now deal largely with human relationships. These are much more difficult to handle than the large-scale relations of society (17, pp. 575-581).

Such emphasis upon the individual citizen, his personal health and welfare, is not so great yet in the underdeveloped areas. But it must come. This means the need for a much closer exploration of the medico-social field, much greater attention to the close relation between health and the social and economic conditions of a community. Here the analytic and evaluative work of social anthropologists and other students of comparative social structures and social values can be of much use to the medical worker. But much more research is needed. There is a great problem of integration to be met, and understanding of its principles can be achieved, as Linton said, only by studying it in process.

REFERENCES

1. Adams, Richard N.: On the Effective Use of Anthropology in Public Health Programs. *Human Organization, 13*:5-15, 1954.
2. Ashton, E. H.: A Sociological Sketch of Sotho Diet. *Transactions, Royal Society of South Africa, 27*:147-214, 1939.
3. Banks, Leslie: *Proceedings, The First World Conference on Medical Education,* 1953. London: Oxford University Press, 1954.
4. Chen Shao-Hsing: Population Growth and Social Change. *Bull. Dept. Archaeol. & Anthro. National Taiwan Univ.,* No. 5, May 1955.
5. Davis, Tom and Davis, Lydia: *Doctor to the Islands.* Boston: Little, Brown, 1954.
6. Foster, George M.: Relationship between Theoretical and Applied Anthropology. *Human Organization, 11*:1-16.
7. George, Dorothy: *London in the Eighteenth Century.* London: Kegan Paul, Trench, Trubner, 1930.
8. Hurgronje, Snouck: *The Achehnese.* London & Leyden: Luzac, London & Brill, 1906.
9. Kelly, Isabel: An Anthropological Approach to Midwifery Training in Mexico. WHO Session, *Nursing and Maternal and Child Health.*
10. Loomis, Charles P. et al.: *Turrialba: Social Systems and the Introduction of Change.* Glencoe: Free Press, 1953.
11. Malcolm, Sheila: *South Pacific Commission Technical Paper,* No. 83, 1955.

12. Paul, Benjamin D., ed.: *Health, Culture and Community.* New York: Russell Sage Foundation, 1955.
13. Phillipps, W. J.: European Influences on Tapu and the Tangi. *J. Polynesian Soc., 63,* 1954.
14. Rapoport, Robert N.; *Changing Navaho Religious Values.* Papers Peabody Museum, Harvard, Vol. 41, No. 2, 1954.
15. Redfield, Robert: *Folk Culture of Yucatan.* Chicago: Chicago University Press, 1941.
16. Saunders, Lyle: *Cultural Difference and Medical Care.* New York: Russell Sage Foundation, 1954.
17. Scheele, Leonard A.: Public Health. *Interrelations Between the Social Environment and Psychiatric Disorders.* New York: Millbank Memorial Fund, 1953.
18. Turbott, I. G.: Diets, Gilbert and Ellice Islands Colony. *J. Polynesian Soc., 58*:36-46, 1949.
19. Uganda Nutrition Committee, *Review,* 1945.
20. Young, Arthur: *Travels in France.* London: George Bell & Sons, 1890.